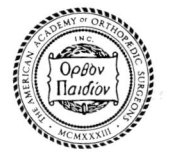

American Academy of Orthopaedic Surgeons
6300 North River Road
Rosemont, Illinois 60018
1-800-626-6726

Legg-Calvé-Perthes Disease

BY

JOHN ANTHONY HERRING, MD
Chief of Staff
Texas Scottish Rite Hospital for Children

Professor, Department of Orthopaedic Surgery
University of Texas Southwestern Medical Center
Dallas, Texas

SERIES EDITOR
Glenn B. Pfeffer, MD

The American Academy of Orthopaedic Surgeons Monograph Series is dedicated to Wendy O. Schmidt, American Academy of Orthopaedic Surgeons senior medical editor, 1987-1991.

LEGG-CALVÉ-PERTHES DISEASE
American Academy of Orthopaedic Surgeons

Legg-Calvé-Perthes Disease
by John Anthony Herring, MD

CONTENTS

PREFACE

In the early part of this century Waldenstrom, Legg, Calvé, and Perthes discovered an interesting little condition involving the hip that was not nearly as destructive as tuberculosis, the condition with which it had been confused. Now, four score and seven years later, we have accumulated enough knowledge to more than fill this monograph. I have intensely studied the clinical aspects of the disorder for the past 12 years and have come to understand and anticipate some of the vagaries of the process. Yet, when a patient appears with a new case of Legg-Calvé-Perthes, it is still difficult to predict that patient's course, plan the appropriate treatment, and know that therapy will be both effective and necessary. Thus, this monograph is published with the hope that sharing our accumulated knowledge will not only assist the clinician in managing children with Legg-Calvé-Perthes, but will also encourage investigators toward further progress in the understanding of the disease.

I would like to thank many individuals who have made this work possible. First, my wife, Kathy, and my daughters for their never-ending support. I must also thank the members of the Legg-Perthes study group who have contributed not just their cases, but their ideas as well in an unselfish attempt to better understand the condition. My secretary, Louise Hamilton, deserves much credit for her work in preparation of the manuscript, as do the members of the media department at Texas Scottish Rite Hospital for Children who prepared all of the visual materials. Finally, I would like to thank Dr. Herbert Kaufer, former member of the Committee on Publications, and Marilyn Fox, PhD, Director of Publications for the Academy, for their help in initiating the monograph. I would also like to thank Joan Abern, Associate Senior Editor in the publications department for her diligent and helpful manuscript editing.

JOHN A. HERRING, MD

LEGG-CALVÉ-PERTHES DISEASE

HISTORY

Legg-Calvé-Perthes disease is an osteochondrosis that affects the capital epiphysis of the femur. This disease, which occurs mainly in boys between the ages of 4 and 12 years, was discovered soon after the advent of the X-ray machine. Imagine the thrill experienced by the muttonchopped physicians of the early Twentieth Century when they first were able to see the bones of a patient. No longer were they limited to a history and physical examination to uncover bone infections, tumors, fractures, and a myriad of other skeletal problems. Roentgen discovered X-rays in 1895, and by 1905, X-ray machines were becoming available to most physicians. As the first decade of the new century waned, a remarkable coincidence of discovery occurred when four surgeons independently recognized a condition that undoubtedly had been present for all of human history. What was the milieu for this discovery, and what were the pertinent observations?

DISCOVERY

The man who probably has the best claim for the first published description of this new disorder was Arthur Legg of Boston. Legg was a quintessential Harvard man; he grew up in Chelsea, Massachusetts, graduated from Harvard college and Harvard Medical School, trained in the Harvard residency programs, and, in fact, even died at the Harvard Club! His interest in this "obscure affliction of the hip joint" began with a boy he first treated at Children's Hospital of Boston for a fracture of the humerus. Two months after the fracture, the boy developed a problem with the hip that was diagnosed as atypical tuberculous coxitis, or as it was then known, "the quiet hip disease."[1] Having observed the development of the disorder from the onset, Legg began to question the nature of the problem and its supposed relationship to tuberculosis. The initial radiographs were equivocal, and subsequent

ones revealed a progression of radiologic changes that did not at all resemble those of tuberculosis. He intuitively suspected these changes were somehow related to deficiency of blood supply.[2] Subsequently, the boy developed the same problem in the other hip. Legg's discovery and review of four similar cases led to his presentation at the American Orthopaedic Association meeting in June 1909 and publication of his paper in February 1910.[1,2]

Meanwhile Jacques Calvé was working as a junior surgeon in Berck-sur-mer, an 1,100 bed French seaside hospital for bone tuberculosis where he had successfully argued for the purchase of an X-ray machine in 1904 or 1905. Calvé led a doctoral candidate named Paul Sourdat to look up 250 of the new radiographs for his thesis because Calvé thought there might be something interesting in all this material. Sourdat found a small number of cases of something that did not seem to behave like tuberculosis of the hip and pointed out this discrepancy in his thesis, which was written in 1909 (Fig. 1).[1] Calvé published his own observations of ten cases in July 1910.[3,4] He noted that the patients did not have much atrophy of the leg and lacked the palpable swelling about the hip characteristic of tuberculosis. The children were not ill, but Calvé felt they were all somewhat rachitic, with two having severe bow legs. Because his radiographs did not reproduce well, he drew the changes he observed, and these detailed drawings rival modern radiographs. Calvé's early awareness of the clinical features was more complete than that of Legg.[1,3,4]

At about the same time, at the polyclinic in Tubingen, Germany, Georg Perthes, a general surgeon with a major interest in bone tuberculosis, wrote (in October 1910) about a disorder that he called "arthritis deformans juvenilis" (Fig. 2).[1,5] These cases had been misdiagnosed as tuberculosis of the hip, and he observed that the course of the disease was much more benign than expected. Perthes described 38 cases, including only five

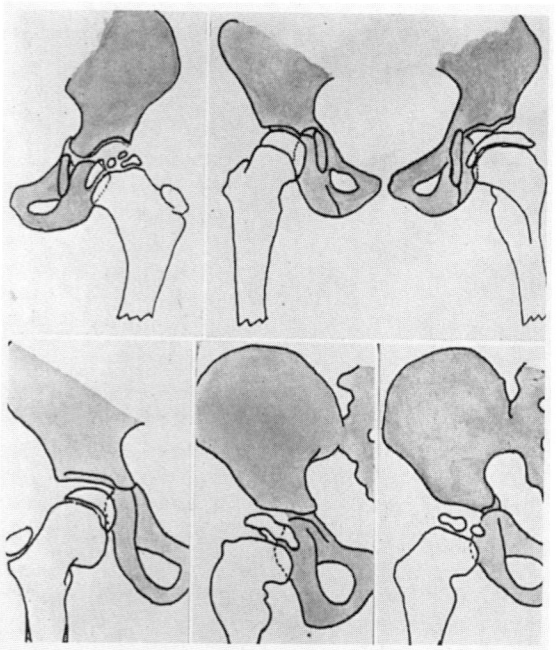

FIGURE 1
Drawings of radiographs made by Paul Sourdat. (Reproduced with permission from Goff CW: *Legg-Calvé-Perthes Syndrome and Related Osteochondroses of Youth.* Springfield, IL, Charles C Thomas, 1954.)

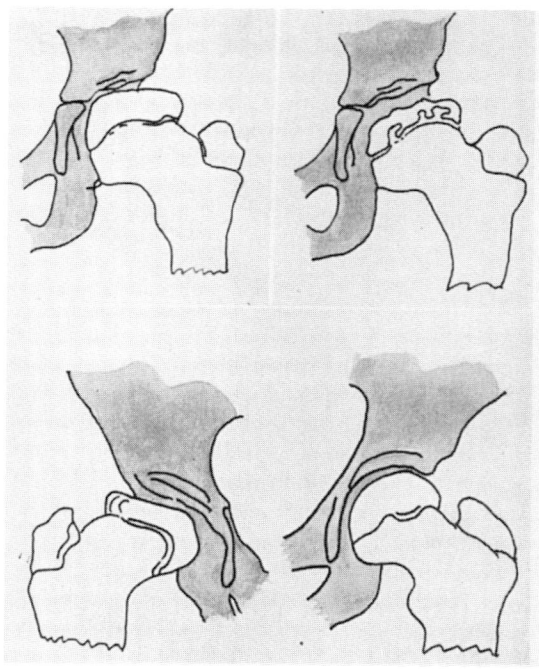

FIGURE 2
Drawings of the radiographic changes noted by Perthes in his original article. (Reproduced with permission from Goff CW: *Legg-Calvé-Perthes Syndrome and Related Osteochondroses of Youth.* Springfield, IL, Charles C Thomas, 1954.)

children younger than 12 years old. He considered the disease to be the youthful variety of adult degenerative arthritis.[5]

There was actually a fourth discoverer (a fifth if one counts Sourdat) of this curious disease. Henning Waldenström of the Karolinska Institute, Stockholm, Sweden, should also be considered one of the pioneers of Legg-Calvé-Perthes disease. In fact, some suggest that it be called Waldenström's disease because he described the radiographic changes a year before the others.[6] His name is not included because, in this early work, Waldenström believed the disease was a form of tuberculosis.[6]

EARLY CONCEPTS

In his original paper,[2] Legg described five patients, noting that the salient features of the disease were an age of onset between 5 and 8 years, a history of an injury, a limp without pain, and little or no spasm or shortening of the extremity. The first patient was treated with traction followed by a splint (probably a patten bottom brace), while three patients were treated in spica

casts. The fifth patient underwent curettage of the femoral neck because of the suspicion of infection. *Staphylococcus* was cultured in an aspirate from one patient, but Legg correctly interpreted this as a contaminant. One boy had incurred an injury in which his legs were hyperabducted, after which he limped for a week and then was asymptomatic for 7 months. Legg hypothesized that the condition could result from an injury that impaired the nutrition (circulation) of the (femoral) head.[2]

In 1916, Legg[7] noted that the patients generally belonged to the "working classes," and he believed this fact favored a traumatic etiology. (Calvé[4] also mentioned that his cases were from the "working class.") Legg pointed out that Hoffa reviewed several cases as a form of juvenile arthritis deformans. The review was published in Deutsche Medizin in 1907. He noted that Freiberg[8] reported a similar case as coxa vara adolescentium in 1905. Legg also asserted that his description preceded that of Calvé by a year, and that Calvé thought the disorder was related to rickets. He presented 55 new cases, noting that the age range was now 2.5 to 12 years, with initial symptoms present for 6 months to 1 year. Twenty-one of his cases were related to trauma, and he found cases in which negative initial radiographs were followed later by avascular changes. For treatment, he suggested a flannel spica for mild cases and a plaster spica cast for more severe cases.[7]

In 1913, Perthes[9] further clarified the clinical features of the disease. He described the disorder as "a self-limiting, non-inflammatory condition, affecting the capital femoral epiphysis with stages of degeneration and regeneration, leading to a restoration of the bone nucleus." Perthes first described the pathology of the disorder, based on a patient who died an accidental death while his hip was in the mid stages of disease evolution. In 1914, Schwarz,[10] a pathologist working with Perthes, originally published his concept of the blood supply of the femoral head, which was quite consistent with data from more modern studies (Fig. 3). Calvé did not publish further on the disorder, but in 1939 wrote an extensive paper on the difference between a Trendelenburg gait and an antalgic gait.[11]

Legg, Calvé, Perthes, and Waldenström were all young men in 1910, when this disorder was described. Legg was 36, Calvé 35, Waldenström 33, and Perthes, the oldest, was 41 years of age. All were beneficiaries of the newly available X-ray machine, and each saw something that had been missed by others. As to who deserves the ultimate credit, there is no sure answer. Legg in 1916 threw his support to Perthes by saying "A new clinical entity has emerged in the category of a juvenile disease affecting the hip. This is very largely due to the work of Dr. Georg Perthes, who...in 1913, presented a classical monograph on the affection in question."[7] Perthes in 1920 wrote a paper about "Legg's Disease" and said that Calvé should be considered the first to report and describe the disease condition. He felt that Legg's article had gone unnoticed (by the Europeans) and had not been reviewed in any other medical journals, and that Legg had not adequately characterized the disease.[12] Sundt stated that Legg had presented his article in Europe in 1910 and pointed out that Waldenström had actually made the first presentation about the disorder. This argument could rage forever, and all these men must obviously share the honor of their discoveries.

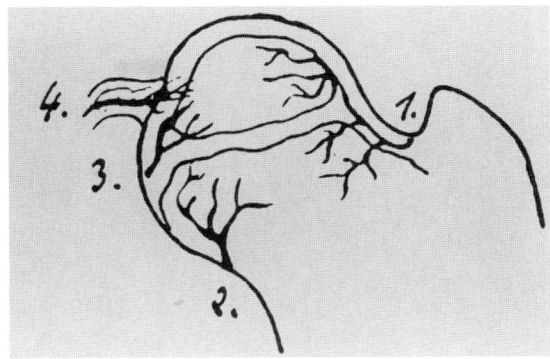

FIGURE 3
Schwarz' drawing of the blood supply of the femoral head. (Reproduced with permission from Schwarz E: A typical disease of the upper femoral epiphysis. *Clin Orthop* 1986;209:5-12.)

TREATMENT

Early

The early treatment concepts for Legg-Calvé-Perthes disease were based on methods used for tuberculous coxitis: bed rest, immobilization, and weight relief. The patten bottom brace was often used. This device suspended the affected leg from an ischial weightbearing caliper and required an elevated shoe on the other foot. Although there was apparent "relief" of direct weightbearing, modern biomechanical studies suggest that the compressive forces of muscles acting across the hip while suspending the leg and brace produce more intra-articular pressure than does simple weightbearing.[13]

In the very early years after the disease was discovered, several of the pioneers expressed serious doubts as to the effectiveness of the popular treatment methods. Calvé[3] stated that the symptoms of the disease rapidly resolved and that he removed any immobilizing apparatus and allowed the patients to walk. In 1927, Legg[14] expressed his doubts, saying, "It must be admitted that while any process which suggests a weakening in bone structure is going on in the hip joint, it would seem theoretically sound treatment to allow no weight-bearing. It has been my experience, however, that relief from weight-bearing has in no way affected the end result." The discussants of this paper disagreed, and Legg replied, "In my cases relief from weight-bearing did not stop the process from going on, and it was kept up for five years."[14] Waldenström,[15] in a 1923 paper, expressed a strong opinion that treatment was ineffective. He noted that "As early as 1909-1910 I had the idea that no intervention should be undertaken.... The prognosis is so good without any treatment whatever and with an operation of the joint we may of course do great harm, even if no effect therefrom is noticed until some long time afterwards.... I believe that treatment should consist in reducing our physical pretensions in respect to the joint, but not so much, however, as to give the child the impression of being weakly." He suggested that during the first 3 to 5 years, the child should not take part in gymnastics, jump on one leg (the diseased one) or jump too much at all, or take very long walks, etc, and that permanent traction with bed rest from 4 to 6 weeks be prescribed as needed for "pains and strong contracture."[15]

Mid Century

These warnings went unheeded, and by the mid 1950s many centers used prolonged recumbency with leg calipers until the femoral head was fully healed radiographically. Pike[16] reported the results of 59 children, who had been tied to a frame in a hospital bed around the clock for periods ranging from 1 to 5 years, claiming to have achieved excellent radiologic results. In those days, many children were hospitalized for 5 or more years, using special carts and gurneys for mobility (Fig. 4). Goff[1] illustrates the prevalent attitudes: "After a few weeks they are privileged to have swimming, and to scoot around the hospital and even the outdoor playground on a low cart which they can propel with their hands. They are allowed to express themselves and to have periods when they can yell and shout, but at the same time the nurses endeavor to instill good manners, consideration of the other fellow, and the type of behavior which their own mothers would desire.... They look forward eagerly to the weekly visits from their parents. Very few remain homesick during their busy, weekly programs."

Goff[17] blazed another trail that turned out to be a dead end. He became intrigued with the fact that the growth rate of cattle could be dramatically increased when they were given Aureomycin (a form of tetracycline). He treated a number of children who had Legg-Perthes with the drug and reported that not only was their growth stimulated, but their disease was ameliorated. This treatment method fell by the wayside

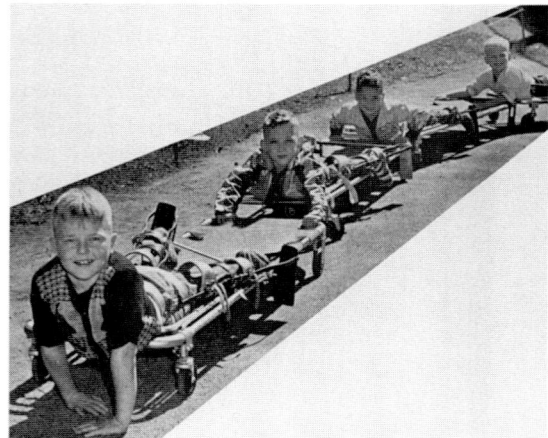

FIGURE 4
Special carts used by children to move about while in the non-ambulatory Newington abduction frames. (Reproduced with permission from Goff CW: *Legg-Calvé-Perthes Syndrome and Related Osteochondroses of Youth.* Springfield, IL, Charles C Thomas, 1954.)

when it was discovered that the mechanism of growth stimulation was related to the flora of the cow's intestine.

Another treatment mode that was popular in the 1950s was the Snyder sling (Fig. 5), which actually was suggested by a parent as a way to get his child to comply with a nonweightbearing prescription.[18] Snyder had no data or results to report; he stated, "Several children are now wearing this type of sling, and are able to walk with crutches and attend orthopedic school. The muscle spasm disappears after a few weeks, and quite normal rounding of the head of the femur results in due time without much atrophy and in most cases with very little shortening."[18]

Current

Most current therapy is based on the containment concept, and the origin of this idea is hard to pinpoint. Harrison and Menon[19] reported treatment with broomstick plasters, which they say were introduced in 1929 (Fig. 6). They pointed out that when the lower limbs are in the anatomic position, the entire femoral head does not fit within the acetabulum; therefore, compression forces will tend to flatten part of the head, leaving the uncovered rim untouched. They noted that the compression would be intense in the ambulatory patient and potent in the supine patient. They said, "Failure to introduce the head completely

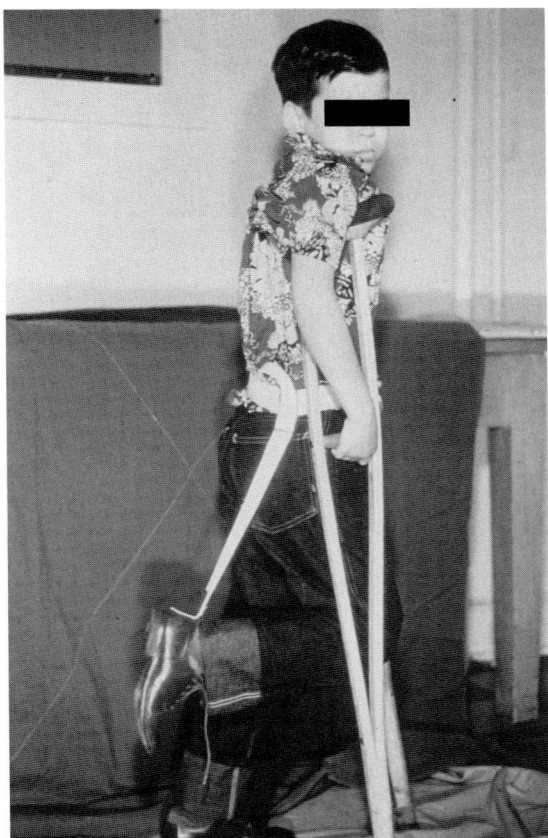

FIGURE 5
A boy wearing a Snyder sling.

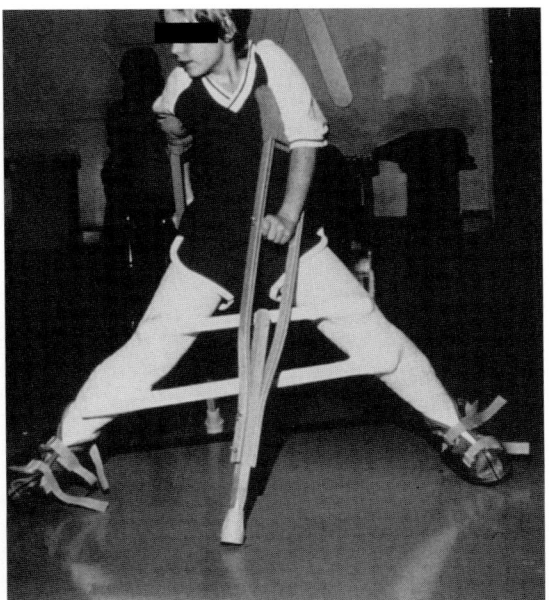

FIGURE 6
Broomstick plasters known as "Petrie casts." The hips are abducted about 45° and the knees slightly flexed. The patient walks by using crutches fore and aft.

into the acetabulum will result in unequal compression of various areas of the epiphysis—high spots and low spots—with resulting deformation. If the head is contained within the acetabular cup, then like jelly poured into a mold the head should be the same shape as the cup when it is allowed to come out after reconstitution." Harrison and associates[20] soon thereafter reported use of ambulatory containment with leather braces that were designed to prevent weightbearing.

Eyre-Brook[21] felt that Legg's pessimism about the effectiveness of treatment was due to "the advanced stage of disease at which treatment is so often begun." He believed treatment should begin while the head is soft but before it becomes deformed, with the aims of maintaining full range of motion and keeping a round head. He stated that the prognosis was relative to the type of disease (cap or mushroom), the age of the patient, the time from onset to treatment, and the effec-

tiveness of the treatment. He believed that progressive deformity resulted from stresses on the femoral head and that treatment must relieve the crushing forces of both weightbearing and muscular contraction. He believed that movement as opposed to immobilization helped round the head, and he recommended traction in bed for 18 to 24 months.

Salter[22] produced avascular necrosis of the femoral head in pigs, and noted that there was a pathologic fracture of the subchondral bone in the early stage of revascularization. He felt this was the time when the head was vulnerable to deformation, and he recommended containment treatment to prevent pressure by the edge of the acetabulum. The containment concept has evolved over the years to include nonsurgical and surgical methods. Although the concept has had many modern detractors, it remains popular but unproven.

Treatment philosophies have continued to evolve over the last two decades. Many who initially recommended containment treatment for all patients have become more selective and treat only those patients judged to be at risk for hip deformity. Brace treatment, which was very widespread in the 1970s, has fewer advocates today.

The enthusiasm for surgical treatment, which was widely used in previous years, has waned considerably over the past decade, and those who still prefer surgery are now more selective. Some have treated patients with measures focused on maintaining the range of motion, while others have opted for symptomatic treatment only. Many modern orthopaedists would probably agree with Eyre-Brook[21] that treatment goals are to maintain a full range of motion and keep the femoral head round, that treatment must relieve the crushing forces of weightbearing and/or muscular contraction, and that movement, as opposed to immobilization, helps round the head.

ETIOLOGY

A great many studies have provided intriguing clues as to the etiology of Legg-Calvé-Perthes disease, but its exact cause is still unknown. Abnormalities of growth and development of affected children have been observed repeatedly, leading to the concept of the "predisposed child."[23-44] Genetic factors have been suggested, but they probably play a minor role, if any.[45-49] Environmental influences have been observed primarily in England, but have not been seen in many other areas.[49-53] Trauma in the predisposed patient also has been implicated.[1,54-56] The pathologic changes in the femoral head are probably the result of vascular events, and various studies have implicated both the arterial and venous systems.[55,57-70] Hematologic abnormalities are known to cause avascular necrosis of bone (osteonecrosis) in patients with such disorders as sickle cell disease, thalassemia, and other coagulopathies, and abnormalities of protein C and S recently have been implicated in Legg-Calvé-Perthes disease.[71-79] Synovitis of the hip occurs early in the disorder and may precede the radiographic changes. Many investigators have studied the incidence of Legg-Calvé-Perthes after synovitis and generally have failed to demonstrate that synovitis has caused the disorder.[80-90]

THE PREDISPOSED CHILD: ABNORMAL GROWTH PATTERNS

Results of many studies have indicated that patients with Legg-Calvé-Perthes disease share certain abnormalities of growth and develop-ment, suggesting that there is a predisposed child, more likely than others to develop the disorder.[23] The most commonly reported abnormality, a delay in the bone age relative to chronologic age, first was reported in 1968.[24,25] The carpal bone age is often 2 or more years behind the chronologic age (Fig. 7) Although the bone age is delayed in the early years of the disease, there later is an acceleration of maturation, which allows the bone age to catch up with the chronologic age. Bohr[26] found that in boys diagnosed before 5 years of age the bone-age delay increased over the subsequent 4 to 5 years while in those diagnosed after 8 years of age the delay decreased over the next few years. Kristmundsdottir and associates[27] noted a radiologic standstill in the bone age with certain carpals more delayed than others. Harrison and associates[28] used the term "skeletal standstill" for the same phenomenon. The capitate and hamate were not delayed, whereas the triquetral and lunate were markedly delayed. Patients with bilateral disease had more delay of the trapezoid than those with unilateral disease.[27] The carpals were more delayed than the radius and ulna, and in bilateral disease, the onset of ossification in the carpals was later than in unilateral disease.[29] Although there is uncontested evidence that most of the children with Legg-Calvé-Perthes disease have distinct abnormalities of bone maturation, the exact relationship to the pathogenesis of the disorder remains unknown.

Exner and Schreiber[30] found that following the period of growth retardation there was a period of excessive compensatory growth that was mirrored in the rate of skeletal maturation. Others found that when stature was plotted against chronologic age, most were in the low-normal percentiles. By studying the children as they grew, the authors found that soon after diagnosis there was a phase of retarded growth velocity, which was followed by a period of catch-up growth. The onset of puberty was normal, and by 12 to 15 years of age the stature and bone age were normal.[29] Cannon and associates[31] noted that boys with diagnosis of Legg-Calvé-Perthes before 6 years of age had an early pubertal growth spurt that was not sustained. Wynne-Davies and Gormley[32] observed that children were undersized at the time of developing Legg-Calvé-Perthes disease and remained shorter than average throughout life. They stated that, "The child who is going to develop Perthes'

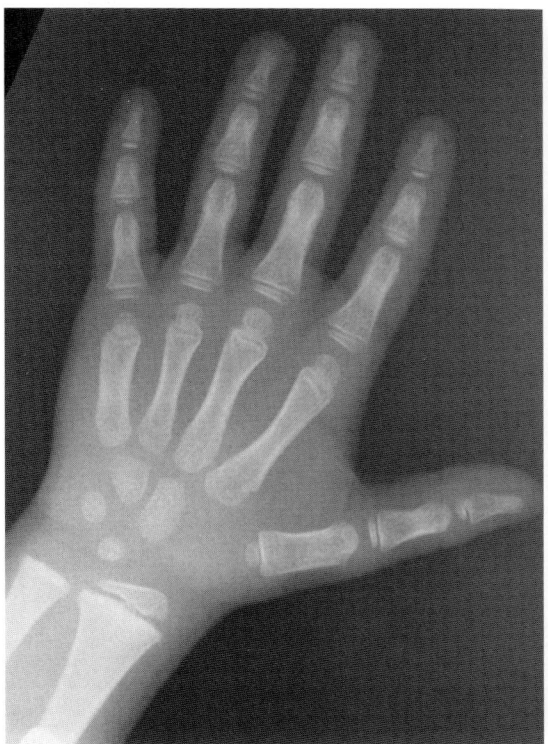 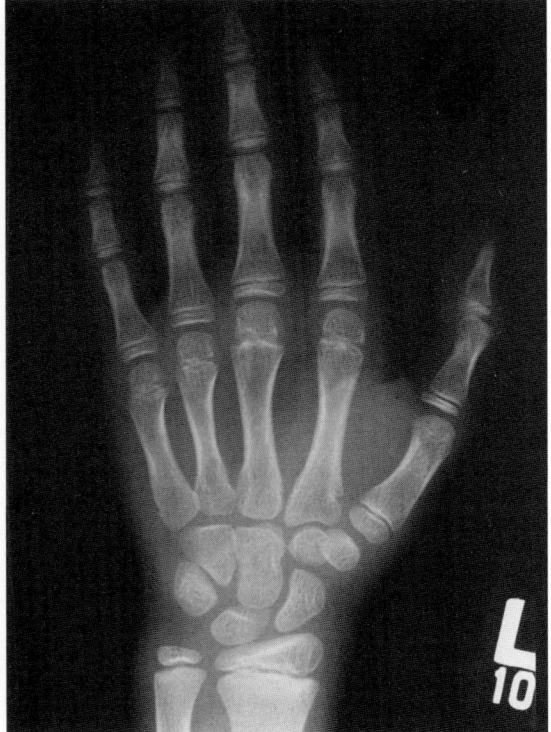

FIGURE 7
Left, This radiograph was taken at the onset of Legg-Calvé-Perthes disease in a boy of 6 years 6 months of age. The bone age is 4 years. **Right,** In a subsequent radiograph of the same patient taken at the chronological age of 12 years, the bone age was read as 11 years 6 months.

disease is already constitutionally and socially at a disadvantage, and during the perinatal period and the first few years of life is perhaps more susceptible to trauma than is a normal child." Why they supposed that the trauma occurred so early is not clear. Hall and associates[33] showed that the children with Legg-Calvé-Perthes disease had smaller hands and feet than either their siblings or a control group.

The abnormal growth patterns of children with Legg-Calvé-Perthes may relate to abnormalities of growth hormone. Tanaka and associates[34] found that somatomedin A was significantly reduced in children with Legg-Calvé-Perthes disease compared to age-matched controls. Motokawa[35] found plasma somatomedin C levels to be lower than normal. His patients were of short stature and had immature bone ages. Neidel and associates[36] expanded on these findings, noting that while normal children had an increase in plasma somatomedin C with age, patients with

Legg-Calvé-Perthes had no such increase in the early stages of the disease. These reports are contradicted by a report by Kitsugi and associates,[37] who found normal somatomedin C activity as measured by radioimmunoassay in children with Legg-Calvé-Perthes disease. Although a number of studies have shown children with Legg-Calvé-Perthes disease to have normal thyroid function, a recent report by Neidel and associates[38] has shown increased plasma levels of free thyroxin and triiodothyronine in children with the disorder.[39,40] The hormonal levels in these children were elevated compared to a control group but remained within the limits of normal.

Another signal for possible systemic abnormalities of the children who have this disorder is the presence of subtle abnormalities of the contralateral hip. Arie and associates[41] noted that the contralateral hip was less round than in controls, with flattening anteriorly and laterally. Harrison and Blakemore[42] found that there was flattening or dimpling of the "normal head" in 48% of cases. Ippolito[43] studied femoral head biopsies and found abnormal cartilage, which surrounded occluded nutrient vessels of the femoral head. He believed, along with Ponseti,[44] that the cartilage abnormalities were part of a systemic abnormality of cartilage metabolism.[43]

GENETIC FACTORS

A genetic etiology has been postulated, but most studies have shown little genetic effect. Wynne-Davies and Gormley[32] reviewed 310 patients with Legg-Calvé-Perthes disease and found no evidence of a genetic factor. No parents were affected, 1.6% of siblings had the disorder, and second and third degree relatives were affected at the rate of the general population. They pointed out that other studies, which show a high familial incidence of the disorder, may have inadvertently included patients with familial epiphyseal dysplasias. Harper and associates[45] reported a mating of affected individuals who had monozygotic twins concordant for Perthes. They found a risk in siblings of less than 1% and a risk of children of an affected parent to be 3%, and they concluded that there was a relatively minor genetic component to the disease.

Other authors believe that there is a genetic factor involved. Hall[46] found evidence for a multifactorial inheritance pattern, with a ratio of 35:4:4:1 for first, second, third, and fourth degree relatives. Burch and Nevelos[47] reviewed a personal series and six other published series and concluded that there was an x-linked recessive factor and an autosomal homozygous allele in each genotype of the disorder. O'Sullivan and associates[48] reported a family with four members with the disorder, but was uncertain whether this represented hereditary or environmental factors. Hall and associates[49] found a higher than normal incidence of minor congenital abnormalities with Legg-Calvé-Perthes disease. These abnormalities included hemivertebrae, deafness, Rubenstein Taybe syndrome, imperforated anus, pyloric stenosis, epilepsy, congenital heart disease, undescended testicle, and short tibia. Their findings may be interpreted to support either a genetic or environmental etiology.[49]

ENVIRONMENTAL FACTORS

Environmental factors may play a role in the etiology of Legg-Calvé-Perthes disease. Several studies document a particularly high incidence of the disorder in certain urban areas of Great Britain. Hall and associates[33,50,51] found a high incidence of the disorder in the inner city area of Liverpool. The affected children were noted to have reduced sitting height and smaller feet than the control group. The incidence was also highest in the lower social classes, and these authors suspected a nutritional etiology. Hall and associates[52] subsequently found low blood manganese levels in the Liverpool children with Legg-Calvé-Perthes disease. Other correlations included being in a lower social class, living in a council house, having parental unemployment, and a larger family. These findings were felt to indicate a nutritional etiology.[53]

TRAUMA

Trauma has been frequently proposed as an etiologic factor, possibly precipitating the osteonecrosis in predisposed individuals. Douglas and Rang[54] suggest that trauma is important in Perthes as well as in many osteochondroses. Chung's[55] studies of femoral head blood supply demonstrate that the major lateral epiphyseal artery has a narrow passage, which could be vulnerable to traumatic interruption. The fact that these vessels pass through a thick, cartilaginous femoral head would also increase the likelihood of traumatic disruption of the vessels.

The Role of Hyperactivity

Many children with Legg-Calvé-Perthes disease are physically very active, and a significant percentage have true hyperactivity or attention deficit disorder. Loder and associates[56] reported that one third of children in their series had abnormally high scores in profiles associated with attention deficit hyperactivity disorder. Hersey found that 43 of 68 children treated with recumbency were extremely hyperactive as they grew up and described them as children who were frequently falling, climbing, and were in constant motion.[1] The extremely active nature of these children may play an as yet undefined role in the etiology of the disorder.

Vascular Factors

Arterial Infarction The final common pathway to the pathologic changes of Legg-Calvé-Perthes disease is the vascular supply to the femoral head. Chung[55] studied 150 specimens of the upper femur from autopsied fetuses and children from 26 weeks of gestation to 14 years of age and described two anastomotic arterial rings around the femoral neck that form the major blood supply of the capital epiphysis (Fig. 8). The extracapsular ring is formed by the medial and lateral femoral circumflex arteries, with most of the blood supply coming from the medial circumflex. Especially important is the lateral portion of the arterial ring, the terminal branch of the medial femoral circumflex, which is the major arterial supply to the femoral head. This vessel pierces the lateral capsule in the posterior trochanteric fossa and becomes the lateral ascending cervical artery. The vessel passes through a narrow passage between the trochanter and the capsule, an area that was especially constricted in children less than 8 years old. There is an intracapsular ring, which is subsynovial and connects four ascending cervical arterial groups. This ring was incomplete in 57% of male and 31% of Chung's female specimens. No vessels usually cross the epiphyseal plate, and there is little blood supply from the ligamentum teres.[55] Catterall and associates[57] studied six femoral heads and five core biopsies of patients with Legg-Calvé-Perthes disease, and the findings ranged from ischemic arrest without infarction to multiple complete infarctions of the epiphyseal bone.

Inoue and associates[58] in 1976 suggested that two infarcts were necessary to produce Legg-Calvé-Perthes disease. In their experiment, two separate infarctions of the femoral head of puppies spaced 4 weeks apart produced changes similar to the human disorder, whereas one infarct failed to reproduce the typical changes. They then studied biopsy specimens of 51 patients and found that 51% had changes characteristic of double infarctions (Fig. 9).

Technetium scanning has proven a useful tool in studying the blood supply of the femoral head in patients with Legg-Calvé-Perthes disease.

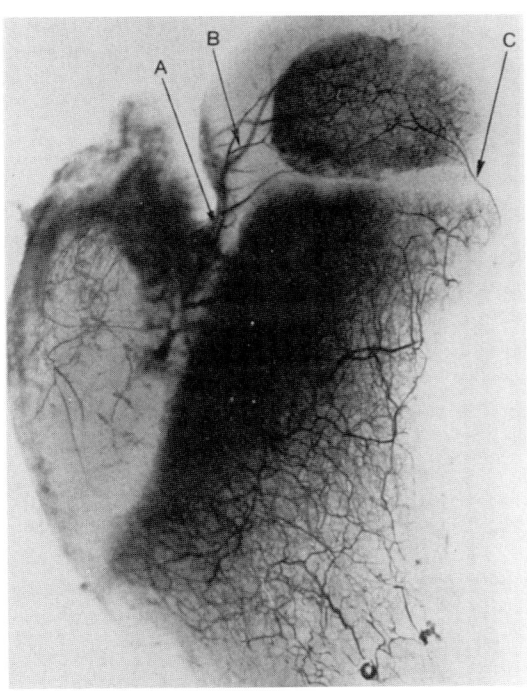
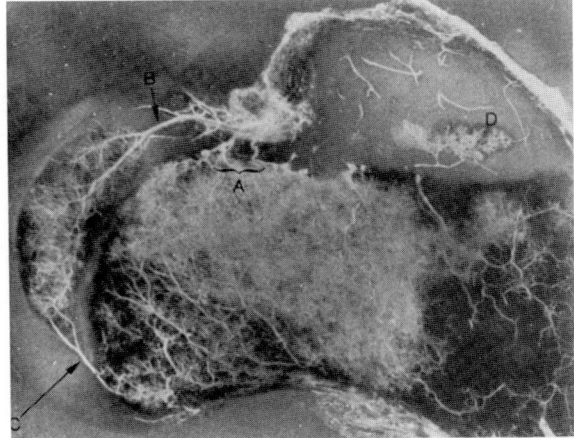

FIGURE 8

The blood supply of the femoral head. **Left,** The lateral ascending cervical artery (A) and the epiphyseal branches of both the lateral (B) and medial (C) ascending cervical arteries as they pass through the perichondrial ring and not the epiphyseal plate. **Right,** The metaphyseal branches (A) of the lateral ascending cervical artery, the epiphyseal branches of the lateral (B) and medial (C) ascending cervical arteries, and the trochanteric ossification center (D) just beginning to form. (Reproduced with permission from Chung SM: The arterial supply of the developing proximal end of the human femur. *J Bone Joint Surg* 1976;58A:961-970.)

Wingstrand and associates[59] used scintigraphy to study 25 children with transient synovitis of the hip. Four of these had decreased uptake initially, but three of the four had normal or increased flow when studied 6 weeks later. The one child who had a persistent defect in blood flow later developed Legg-Calvé-Perthes disease. Their interpretation was that some children who are brought in with transient synovitis have transient ischemia of the femoral epiphysis, and some of these have more severe or recurrent episodes of ischemia so that they develop Legg-Calvé-Perthes disease.[59] Rutskii and associates'[60] scans showed decreased uptake of radioisotope in the upper pole of the femoral head along with reduced blood flow in the femoral artery on the affected side in the early stage of the disease, even before there were radiographic changes.

Angiography has also been used to study children with Legg-Calvé-Perthes disease. Theron[61] performed angiography of the femoral head in 11 cases and found definite obstructions of the superior capsular arteries in the first 5 months after the onset of symptoms. Studies later in the disease process showed revascularization. In one patient, decreased flow with the hip extended improved when the hip was flexed to 30°.[61] Another group performed angiography in 30 patients and found a general decrease of blood flow, along with a major decrease in flow of the medial circumflex artery (Fig. 10).[62] O'Hara and Dommisse[63] studied black African children and found that the largest contribution to the blood supply of the femoral head was from the inferior gluteal artery. They suggested that this variation may explain the rarity of Legg-Calvé-Perthes in black children. Fujikawa[64] compared the blood supply of the femoral head in small dogs, which tend to spontaneously develop osteonecrosis, to that in normal sized mongrels. The most distinct difference between the two species was in the channel of the superior retinacular vessels. In miniature dogs, these vessels go through the shallow neck and appear as a suspended bridge. In normal sized mongrels, they go through the deep fossa of the femoral neck and appear to be better protected.[64]

Abnormal Venous Drainage Abnormalities of venous drainage of the femoral head and neck have also been well documented, especially in studies from Japan. A number of authors have documented elevated venous pressures in the

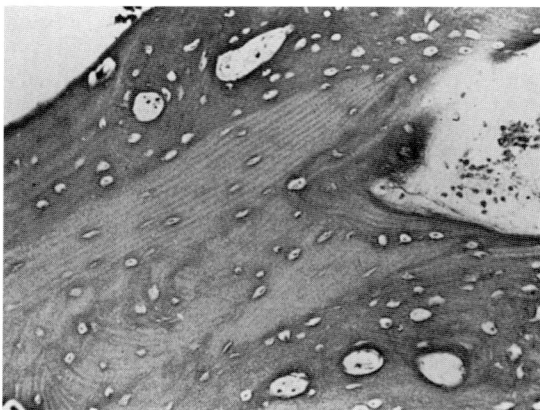

FIGURE 9
Pathological specimen showing dead lamellar bone with a thick surface layer of dead woven bone, 14 months after the onset of symptoms. (Reproduced with permission from Inoue A, Freeman MA, Vernon-Roberts B, et al: The pathogenesis of Perthes' disease. *J Bone Joint Surg* 1976;58B:453-461.)

affected femoral necks associated with venous congestion in the metaphysis.[65-69] Venous drainage, which normally exits via the medial circumflex vein, goes more distally into the diaphyseal veins. Heikkinen and associates[70] found that these abnormalities of venous flow were present in the almost all the children (46 of 55 hips) in the initial and fragmentation stages, and in just less than half of the hips in the restitution stage. In the healed stage, the venous flow was normal. They also found that hips with the most severe radiographic changes had the most disturbed venous drainage (Fig. 11).[70]

Venous obstruction may be either an etiologic factor or a response to some other event. Liu and Ho[65] believed it to be etiologic. They were able to produce osteonecrosis in a dog model by obstructing venous drainage and elevating intraosseus pressure by injecting silicone into the femoral neck. At this point, the venous abnormalities are established as a consistent finding, but whether this represents an etiologic or secondary factor remains to be proven.

Abnormal Coagulation Avascular necrosis of the femoral head is common in patients with hemoglobinopathies, such as sickle cell disease and thalassemia,[71-73] and has also been seen in patients with leukemia, lymphoma, idiopathic thrombocytopenic purpura, and hemophilia.[74-77] Hyperviscosity of the blood was found in children

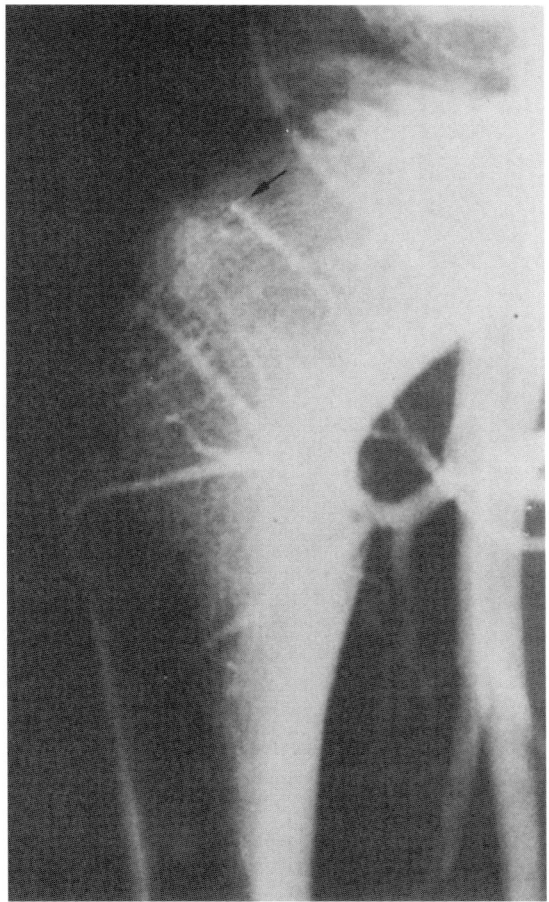

FIGURE 10
An arteriogram showing interruption of the medial circumflex artery (arrow). (Reproduced with permission from de Camargo FP, de Gre Jr, Tovo R: Angiography in Perthes' disease. *Clin Orthop* 1984;191:216-220.)

with Legg-Calvé-Perthes disease by Kleinman and Bleck,[78] but other studies did not confirm this finding. Abnormalities of the clotting mechanisms as represented by deficiencies of protein C and S and by the presence of hypofibrinolysis were found in a recent study.[79] In this study, Glueck and associates[79] studied eight patients with Legg-Calvé-Perthes disease and found that five had abnormalities of venous thrombus formation. They also found that affected family members had a history of other thrombotic events. In a further study, Glueck and associates[80] found that of 44 children with Legg-Calvé-Perthes disease, 23 had thrombophilia, 19 with protein C deficiency, and four with protein S deficiency; seven had high lipoprotein (a); and three had hypofibrinolysis. By comparison, the incidence of protein S and C deficiencies in the general population is only 1/15,000. These findings, if confirmed, suggest a mechanism for thrombotic venous occlusion as the etiology of the Legg-Calvé-Perthes disease.

SYNOVITIS

What is the role of synovitis in this disorder? Do children with synovitis from miscellaneous causes develop osteonecrosis as a result of intracapsular pressure, or is synovitis simply the first manifestation of the hip pathology? From the many studies that have been done, it can be concluded that synovitis is often the first symptom of Legg-Calvé-Perthes, but that rarely, if ever, does synovitis cause the disease. For example, Kallio and associates[81] followed 119 children after transient synovitis and none developed Legg-Calvé-Perthes disease. Sharwood[82] followed 101 children, and only two developed subsequent Legg-Calvé-Perthes disease. Mukamel and associates[83] followed 455 cases of transient synovitis and found that 17 developed radiographic changes of Legg-Calvé-Perthes disease. They noted that those who developed Perthes remained symptomatic, while symptoms in the others resolved, suggesting that synovitis is the first symptom of the disease. Haueisen and associates[84] performed a 30-year review of 497 cases of synovitis and found three who developed Legg-Calvé-Perthes, two who had juvenile arthritis, and one osteoid osteoma. Nineteen cases had recurrence of the synovitis. Landin and associates[85] found 10 cases of Legg-Calvé-Perthes out of 294 cases of synovitis. Mallet and associates[86] followed 38 children and found that one third of them had subsequent radiographic changes that resembled the mildest form of Legg-Calvé-Perthes disease.

Many children with synovitis can be found to have abnormalities of femoral head circulation in the acute phase of the synovitis. Although this would suggest that osteonecrosis will follow, the circulation returns to normal in most of them and they do not develop Legg-Calvé-Perthes disease. Pay and associates[87] studied three children with synovitis who had low signal patterns on T1-weighted magnetic resonance imaging (MRI) images suggesting osteonecrosis. All three returned to normal and the symptoms resolved. They suggested that this represented transient bone marrow edema. Houben and associates[88]

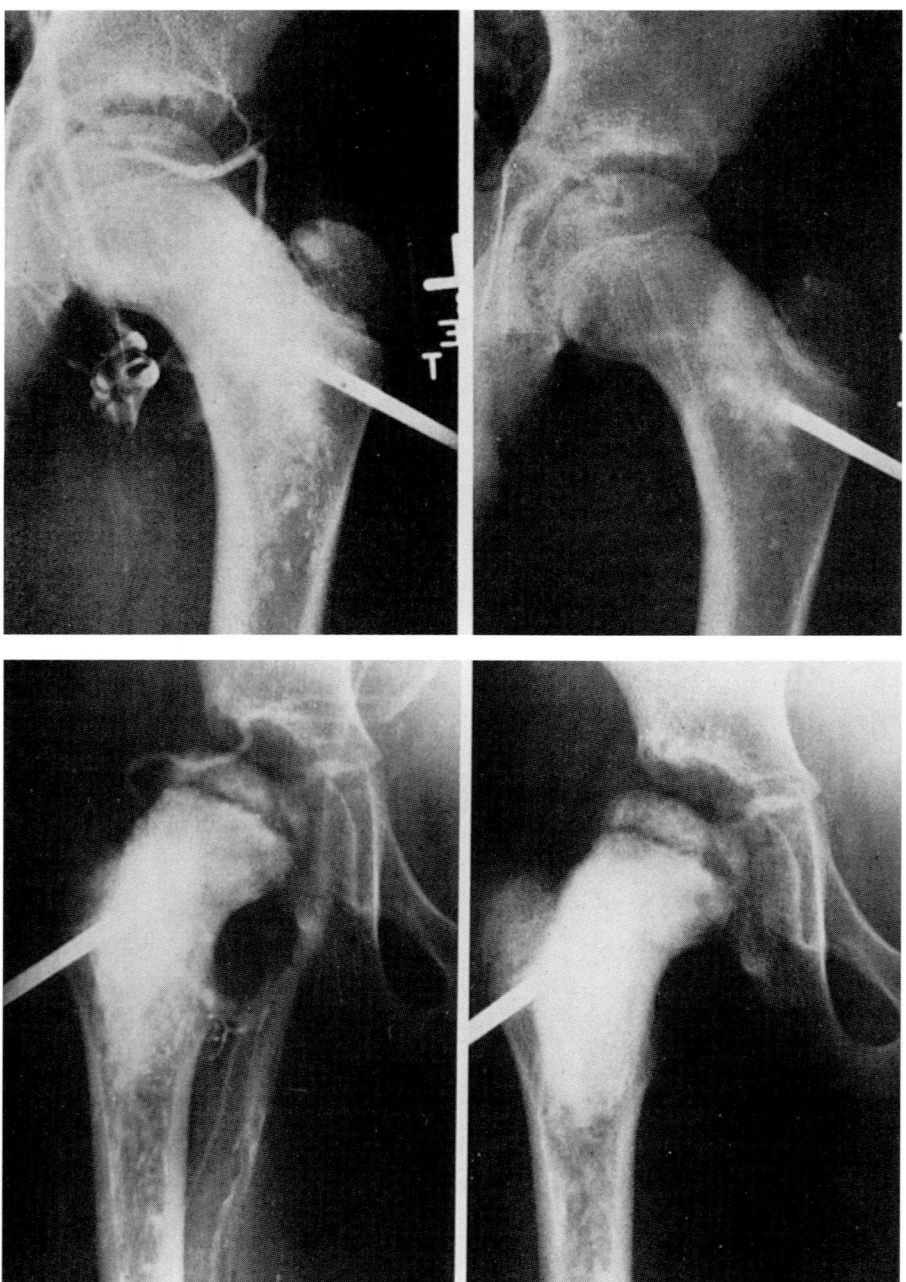

FIGURE 11

Top, Venogram of a normal hip. **Left,** Immediately after injection of 5 ml of contrast medium. The gluteal veins are present and normal. The ischial, medial circumflex, and lateral circumflex veins are well visualized, and there is no diaphyseal reflux of the contrast medium. **Right,** The contrast material is almost completely cleared 5 minutes after injection. **Bottom,** Venogram from an affected hip. **Left,** Immediately after injection of contrast medium, the gluteal and medial circumflex veins are absent. The lateral circumflex vein is seen, as are numerous nutrient veins. There is marked diaphyseal reflux of the contrast material. **Right,** Five minutes after injection of the contrast material, the radiograph shows the persistence of a considerable amount of contrast material within the femoral neck and shaft. (Reproduced with permission from Green NE, Griffin PP: Intra-osseous venous pressure in Legg-Perthes disease. *J Bone Joint Surg* 1982;64A:666-671.)

performed dynamic scintigraphy in 30 children with synovitis. Sixty-three percent had decreased isotopic activity during the early stages of arterial filling of the head. Eight days later only 23% had asymmetry, and 15 days later only three remained abnormal. Two of these three developed Legg-Calvé-Perthes disease.[88] Wingstrand and associates[59] studied 25 cases and found four with markedly abnormal uptake of isotope. At 6 weeks, three were normal and the fourth remained abnormal and developed Legg-Calvé-Perthes disease. Finally, Glefand and associates[89] studied nine children with synovitis, slipped capital epiphysis, hemarthrosis, and postdislocation and found that all had loss of isotope uptake initially. Six of these children revascularized fully, and three had subsequent changes of osteonecrosis.

In patients with synovitis, the position of the hip has been studied relative to intra-articular pressure. In extension and internal rotation, the intra-articular pressures were found to be elevated to several times systolic blood pressure.[90] Kallio and Ryöppy[91] studied 94 hips with synovitis and found that in early Legg-Calvé-Perthes the pressures were mildly elevated. Patients with idiopathic synovitis had moderately elevated pressures, and those with septic arthritis had very high pressures. Extension and internal rotation raised the pressure from 2.3 to 26 kPa, suggesting that immobilization or traction should always be in a position of at least 30° of hip flexion.

PATHOLOGY

Even though Legg-Calvé-Perthes disease is not a fatal affliction, and almost no surgery is done directly on the femoral head, a number of pathologic specimens have been examined. Perthes[9] in 1913 described a femoral head from the necropsy of a boy who died an accidental death. Schwarz working with Perthes also described a pathologic specimen in 1913 and suggested that the pathologic findings were due to loss of blood flow (Fig. 3).[11]

Catterall and associates[57] reported on the pathology obtained from six necropsy specimens, five core biopsies, and five normal controls. They found that the articular cartilage was thicker than normal in both the affected and the unaffected femoral heads. In the unaffected hip, the growth plate was thinner than normal, with irregular cell columns and primary spongiosa. The affected head had greater interference with ossification along the growth plate, with columns of cartilage stretching unossified into metaphyseal region. In one group, changes were found mainly in the anterior part of the head (Fig. 12).

The pathology of the bony epiphysis showed necrotic trabeculae, a thickened subchondral bone plate, and necrotic marrow. Catterall and associates[57] noted that new bone was formed appositionally on the surface of necrotic trabeculae, and vascular tissue was found in the periphery of the head. In specimens where the disease had gone on longer there was more vascular tissue similar to an immature fracture callus. In some specimens there were thickened trabeculae with successive layers of bony apposition but no bone necrosis. The radiolucent areas of these mildly involved heads were composed of fibrocartilage with no active ossification.[57]

Four varieties of metaphyseal changes have been found. First, there was an excess of fatty marrow. Second, circumscribed osteolytic lesions with a sclerotic margin were observed. A third finding was a widened growth plate with disorganized ossification and with columns of unossified cartilage streaming down into the metaphysis. The fourth change was extension of the growth plate down the side of femoral neck. Catterall and associates[57] felt that the metaphyseal lucencies seen radiographically represented unossified cartilage from the growth plate. The pathologic findings, especially those of the uninvolved hip, indicated to them that this is a systemic disease. In the mildest type of disease, they believed there was probably interruption of blood supply insufficient to infarct but enough to disrupt growth and ossification. They postulated two episodes of infarction in the middle groups and repeated infarctions in the final group.

Ponseti and associates[92] studied biopsy specimens of the lateral femoral head and neck from five patients. Beneath the normal articular cartilage there was a thick zone of hyaline (epiphyseal) cartilage containing sharply demarcated areas of hypercellular and fibrillated cartilage with prominent blood vessels (Fig. 13). Ultrastructural examination of these areas revealed many irregularly oriented large collagen fibrils and variable amounts of proteoglycan granules. The investigators found in the fibrillar area a high proteoglycan

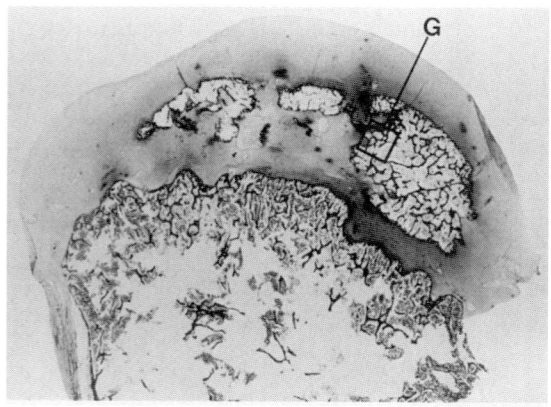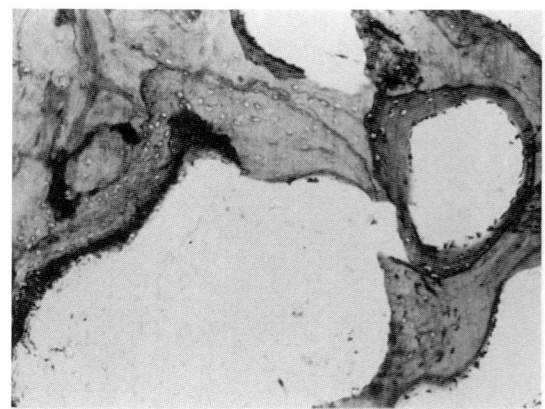

FIGURE 12

A pathologic specimen from Catterall. **Left,** There is considerable thickening of the articular cartilage, which is perforated by a vessel supplying the epiphysis. The central dense area has been completely replaced by a fibrocarilaginous material. The trabecular bone on the medial and lateral aspects shows extensive avascular necrosis as does the bone formed by endochondral ossification on the deep surface of the articular cartilage. **Right,** High power of area G (left) showing grossly thickened trabeculae with extensive avascular necrosis. The many cement lines suggest recurrent episodes of remodeling. The marrow is viable and there is appositional new bone formation on the surface of the avascular trabeculae. (Reproduced with permission from Catterall A, Pringle J, Byers PD, et al: A review of the morphology of Perthes' disease. *J Bone Joint Surg* 1982;64B:269-275.)

content, a decrease in structural glycoproteins, and a different size of collagen fibrils from that of normal epiphyseal cartilage. The lateral physeal margin was often irregular, with a marked reduction of collagen and proteoglycan granules, and it contained numerous large lipid inclusions. They postulated that this is localized expression of a generalized, transient disorder of epiphyseal cartilage with changes similar to those seen in the vertebral end plates in patients with juvenile kyphosis. They believe that this epiphyseal change is primary, and that the collapse and necrosis of the femoral head could result from the breakdown and disorganization of the matrix of the epiphyseal cartilage, followed by abnormal ossification.[92]

Inoue and associates[58] produced a Perthes-like disorder in puppies by inducing two infarcts separated by a 4-week period of time. They then studied 57 human biopsy specimens, and just over half of the specimens showed characteristic changes of double infarction separated by a time interval. The cardinal finding was that of dead woven bone overlaying dead trabecular bone (Fig. 9). They concluded that typical Legg-Calvé-Perthes disease was due to infarction repeated over some time interval.[58]

Mickelson and associates[93] compared the pathologic changes in naturally occurring osteonecrosis in dogs with those of Legg-Calvé-Perthes disease. They concluded that the flattening of the femoral head is the result of mechanical collapse, asymmetric growth, and disturbed enchondral ossification at the growth plate.

CLINICAL FEATURES

Sundt wrote an excellent description of the clinical features of Legg-Calvé-Perthes disease in 1920. He observed that the disorder arises in childhood between the second and twelfth years of life, with the peak ages being between 6 and 8 years. He found that boys were affected four times as often as girls, and 10% of cases were bilateral. He also noted some familial accumulation and believed that trauma often initiated the symptoms. His patients usually presented with a limp and some had pain in the hip, thigh, or knee. Symptoms were often low grade, and considerable time elapsed before the patient saw a doctor. The main physical finding was limitation of range of motion of the hip, especially abduction and internal rotation, and also there usually was mild atrophy of the femoral muscles. These observations agree with modern observations. For example, in 1982 Catterall[94] found that the mean age at onset was 6 years, 82% of children were between 4 and 9 years old, and boys developed the disorder 3.7 times as often as girls.

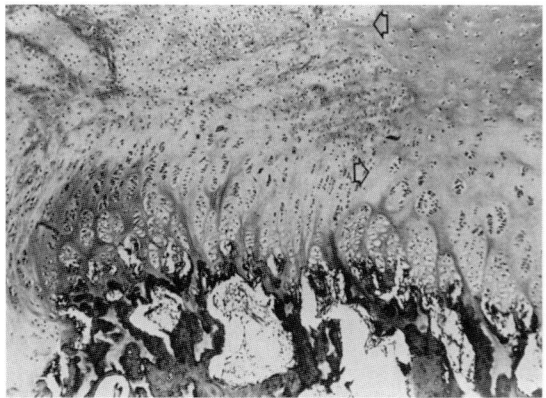

FIGURE 13
A high magnification of the peripheral part of the physis. In the lateral two thirds of this figure, the resting zone is very abnormal, with numerous chondrocytes and a fibrillated matrix. Beneath the abnormal cartilage, the physis is poorly organized and the ossification is irregular. The borderline between normal and abnormal cartilage is well delineated (arrows). (Reproduced with permission from Ponseti IV, Maynard JA, Weinstein SL, et al: Legg-Calvé-Perthes disease: Histochemical and ultrastructural observations of the epiphyseal cartilage and physis. *J Bone Joint Surg* 1983;65A:797-807.)

Waldenström[15] observed that the clinical course was quite variable. He noted that most patients presented with a limp and had slight loss of motion and that there was frequently a history of trauma. He found that a few children got well with a minor change of shape of the femoral head and few symptoms, whereas most had a more severe course, with greater loss of motion, especially abduction and internal rotation, and with pain while walking.

HISTORY

The most frequent presenting complaint is that of a limp, and it is often the parent who first notices it. The limp is worse after activities and improves following periods of rest. Late in the day, after prolonged walking, the limp is more noticeable.

Pain is the second most common complaint. The pain may be located in the groin, anterior hip area, or around the greater trochanter. Referral of pain to the knee is common and may confuse the unwary examiner. The pain usually is worse late in the day and with greater activity, and night pain is frequent. The patient may recall that the limp and pain first began after an injury or very strenuous activity.

The parents and the patient often recall a remote episode of trauma, usually several months earlier, after which the patient had hip pain and a limp. The earlier symptoms usually resolve completely after a few days. The early traumatic event is often a fall or twisting injury.

The symptoms may wax and wane, and the patient may voluntarily reduce his or her activity level to alleviate the pain. When the symptoms are mild, the parent often delays many months before seeking medical attention for the child.

Further questioning often reveals that the affected child has an unusually high activity level. He or she is often characterized as constantly in motion, doing more jumping and running than other children. Some of the children also have problems with attention span and are considered pathologically hyperactive, and some receive medication for this.

The parents will also mention that the child is small for his or her age. Thus, the picture often emerges of the smaller, often thin, very active if not hyperactive child, running and jumping all the time, and limping after these activities. This picture occasionally is contradicted by the obese, inactive child with the same disorder.

The family history occasionally is positive for another family member with Legg-Calvé-Perthes, but this is the exception rather than the rule. If there is strong family history of hip abnormalities, especially if bilateral, the disorder is likely to be a familial epiphyseal dysplasia, which may mimic Legg-Calvé-Perthes disease.

PHYSICAL EXAMINATION

The most important rule of physical examination is to remember the value of simple observation. It is useful to observe the activity level of the child, noting, for example, if the child jumps on and off the examination table. The physician should look for scars and signs of other injuries. (It is not too uncommon for a child with Legg-Calvé-Perthes to come in with a cast on his arm from a wrist fracture.)

The child will limp; the limp usually is a combination of an antalgic and a Trendelenburg gait (Fig. 14). The child will try to disguise the limp in the examination room, and the limp will be more apparent when the patient is unaware of being observed. The Trendelenburg test will be positive on the affected side. There often is atrophy of the gluteus, quadriceps, and hamstring muscles,

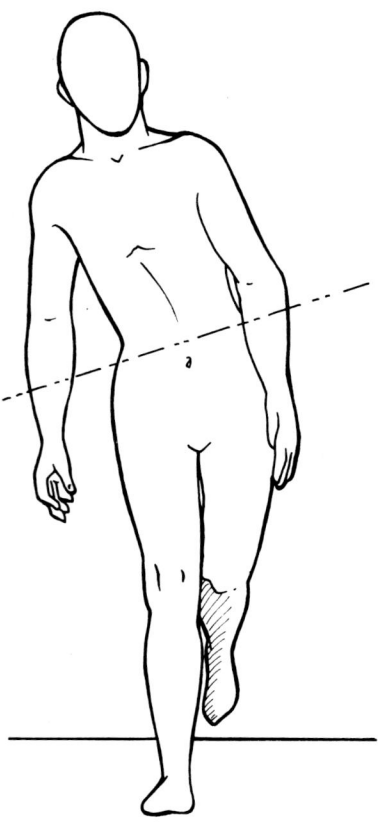

FIGURE 14
A drawing of a child with an abductor limp. In stance phase of gait the person leans the body over the affected hip to reduce the force of the abductor muscles and reduce the pressure within the joint.

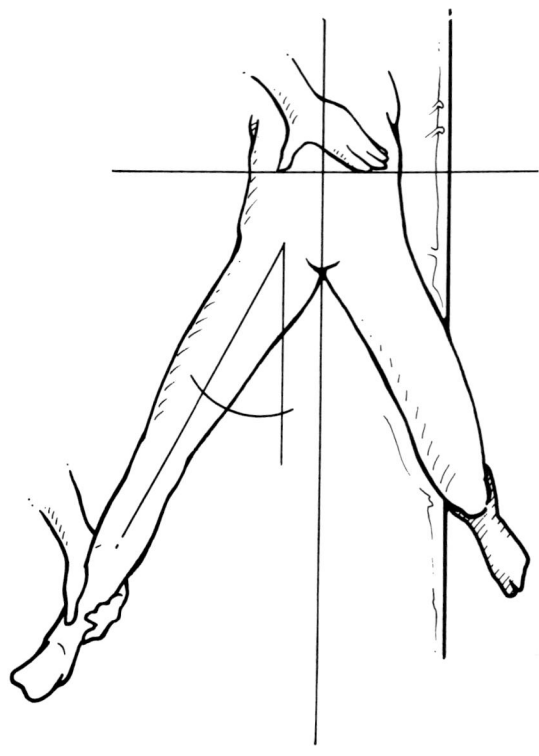

FIGURE 15
To examine for hip abduction, it is helpful to stabilize the pelvis by dropping the unaffected limb over the side of the table.

depending upon the severity and duration of the disorder.

In the early stages of the disease, the restriction of hip motion is variable. In many patients, there may be only minimal loss of motion at the extremes of internal rotation and abduction, and the log roll test will be positive (Fig. 15). In other children, there is a reduction in the range of abduction and internal rotation with the rotational loss best appreciated in the prone position. At this stage there usually is no flexion contracture.

In the early phase of the disease, the loss of motion is caused by muscle spasm. Thus, if the physician examines the hip very gently, a greater range can be demonstrated. Likewise, if the child is examined after a night of bed rest, the range will be much better than later in the day. I recall see-

ing a patient the morning after he was admitted for traction for a stiff hip, commenting to the mother that treatment was obviously having an effect because he had already regained full motion. The mother agreed and mentioned the fact that the child had not yet been placed in traction!

Further into the disease process, the examination may change considerably. Children with mild disease may maintain a minimal loss of motion at the extremes only and subsequently regain full mobility. Those with more severe disease will progressively lose motion, especially abduction and internal rotation. Late cases may have adduction contractures and very limited rotation, but the range of flexion and extension is only rarely compromised.

COURSE OF THE DISEASE
The stages of the disease were well described by Waldenström[95] as set forth in Outline 1. Most

authors have reduced the Waldenström classification to four stages: the initial, fragmentation, healing, and residual stages. In a retrospective study, the interval from the first radiograph taken to the onset of fragmentation was found to be a mean of 6 months (range: 1 to 14 months), while the fragmentation stage lasted 8 months (range: 2 to 35 months). The healing phase (reossification) lasted 51 months (range: 2 to 122 months).[96]

The clinical findings parallel the radiographic stages to some degree. In the early phase of the disease, when there is only increased density of the femoral head radiographically, there may be intermittent exacerbation and relief of symptoms and signs. Periods of minimal pain and limp may be punctuated by periods of discomfort lasting 1 or 2 weeks. In this phase, there is often a subchondral fracture, and clinical worsening may accompany this radiographic finding.[97]

As the hip enters the fragmentation stage, the femoral head will begin to collapse and extrude from the acetabulum. The patient usually has more definite loss of motion at this stage, especially of abduction and internal rotation. Pain and limp are worse at this stage also. Because there is deformation of the femoral head, the range of motion does not return to normal after resting the hip. In more severe cases, the clinical findings gradually worsen throughout the fragmentation stage. In milder cases, there is less change of femoral head shape and the symptoms may be minimal. In the mildest cases, the fragmentation stage is very abbreviated and the patient will have no symptoms.

In the healing phase, which is heralded radiographically by new bone formation in the subchondral areas of the femoral head, the patient usually has few symptoms. Range of motion may remain limited with the degree of loss of motion proportional to the change of shape of the femoral head, but the child has usually returned to full activities without complaints. As the femoral head approaches full reossification, the patient is usually completely asymptomatic.

Children who continue to have pain through the healing phase often have very delayed reossification in the central portion of the femoral head. This soft area in the head may later be the source of a loose fragment or osteochondritis dissecans lesion. The patient will complain of locking and popping, and occasionally crepitance with range of motion can be elicited.

OUTLINE 1

STAGES OF LEGG-CALVÉ-PERTHES DISEASE

I. The evolutionary period: 3 to 4 years
  a. Initial stage: ½ to 1 year;
     a dense epiphysis with lucencies
  b. Fragmentation stage: 2 to 3 years
II. Healing period: 1 to 2 years; epiphysis homogeneous
III. Growing period: to the conclusion of growth
IV. Definite stage

DIFFERENTIAL DIAGNOSIS

The known causes of osteonecrosis include hemoglobinopathies such as sickle cell disease and thalassemia,[71-73] leukemia, lymphoma, idiopathic thrombocytopenic purpura, and hemophilia.[74-77] In most patients these abnormalities can be ruled out with a careful history and physical examination. Black children rarely develop Legg-Calvé-Perthes disease and should have appropriate studies to rule out hemoglobinopathies. Hypothyroidism produces changes that resemble Legg-Calvé-Perthes, and if the radiographic findings are atypical this diagnosis should be considered.[98] Some patients with hypothyroidism have "pseudofragmentations," which are progressive ossification sites in the femoral head, and these sometimes progress to deformity of the head and coxa plana.[99]

Diagnoses of multiple epiphyseal dysplasia and spondyloepiphyseal dysplasia should be considered, especially if there is a strong family history or bilateral disease (Fig. 16).[100] Children with multiple epiphyseal dysplasia and spondylo epiphyseal dysplasia have symmetric flattening, fragmentation, and uniform mild sclerosis of the femoral head and no involvement of the metaphysis.[101] In Legg-Calvé-Perthes disease, however, there is asymmetry of head involvement with areas of increased density, and there are metaphyseal changes.[100,102] Children with epiphyseal dysplasia have short stature and abnormalities of other epiphyses, especially flattening of the distal femoral epiphysis. Bilateral disease in Legg-Calvé-Perthes is usually sequential, with disease developing in one hip a year or more before the second hip, whereas in the epiphyseal dysplasias the hips are involved simultaneously.

Several authors have reported osteonecrosis complicating the changes of epiphyseal dyspla-

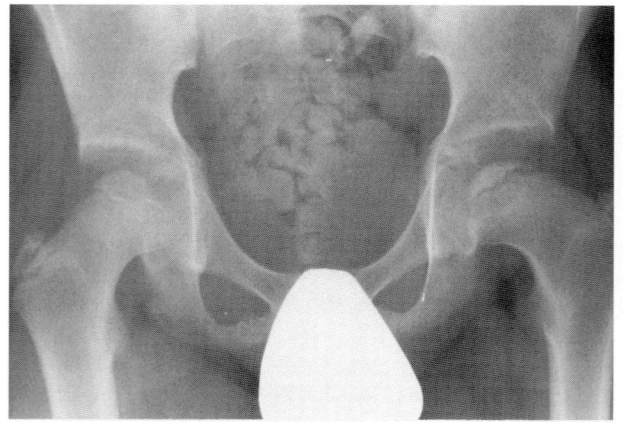
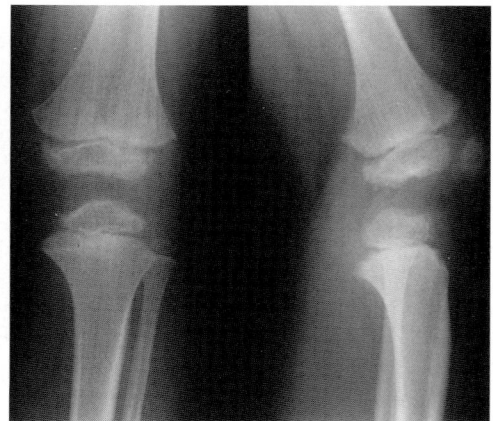
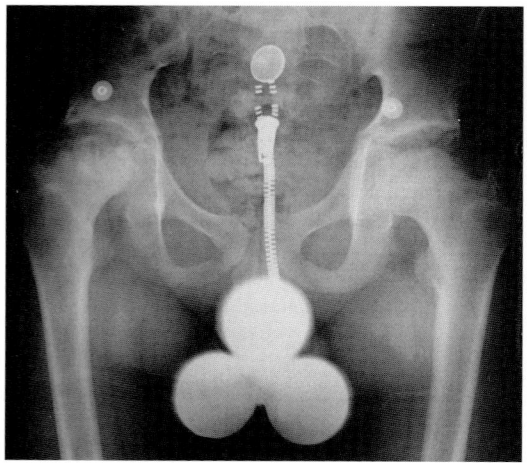
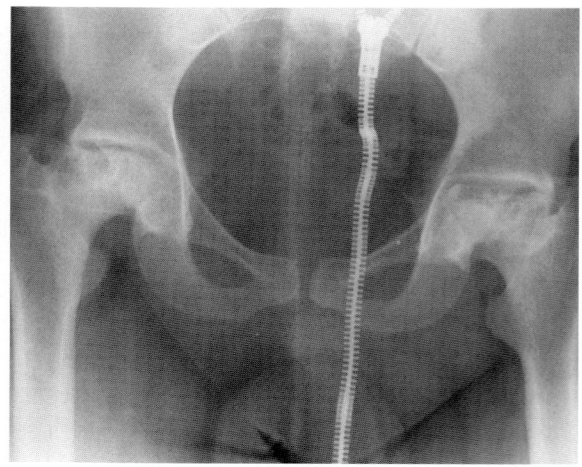

FIGURE 16
A 9-year 7-month old boy who has pain in the hip and whose father had bilateral "Legg Perthes" and was considering total hip replacement at age 40. The diagnosis is multiple epiphyseal dysplasia with an autosomal dominant inheritance pattern, a disorder often mistaken for Legg-Calvé-Perthes disease. **Top left,** Anteroposterior (AP) radiograph showing increased density of the left femoral head and a right femoral head that is smaller than normal. **Top right,** AP and lateral radiographs of the knees showing irregularity of the distal femoral and proximal tibial epiphyses. **Bottom left,** AP radiograph at 13-years 7-months of age. The patient now has bilateral symptoms. There are bilateral irregularities of the femoral heads with more fragmentation now on the right. **Bottom right,** AP radiographs of the patient's father showing bilateral flattening and cystic changes in both femoral heads.

sia.[103] Mandell and associates[104] reported ten patients with multiple epiphyseal dysplasia who also had superimposed changes of avascular necrosis of the femoral head. These changes included sclerosis and subchondral fissuring, which were superimposed on already irregular ossification centers. MRI and scintigraphy confirmed the avascular nature of these changes.

Changes similar to those in Legg-Calvé-Perthes have also been seen in many unusual syndromes. These include Maroteaux-Lamy syndrome,[105]

osteochondroma of the femoral neck,[106] multiple osteochondromatosis,[107] synovial osteochondromatosis,[108] metachondromatosis,[109] and the Schwartz-Jampel syndrome.[110] The tricho-rhino-phalangeal syndrome also produces Perthes-like hip findings.[111,112] The observer should look for abnormal hair, and facies and hand films will show characteristic cone-shaped epiphyses.[113]

Legg-Calvé-Perthes has been reported as late as 5 years after treatment of congenital dislocation of the hip.[114] Coexistent slipped capital femoral epiphysis and Legg-Calvé-Perthes in the same child has also been reported.[115] Osteonecrosis occurs after traumatic hip dislocation, and in younger children it resembles Legg-Calvé-Perthes disease.[116]

At times, there are other radiographic findings that resemble Legg-Calvé-Perthes disease. Ozonoff and Ziter[117] described the femoral head notch, a normal variant that often is mistaken for Legg-Calvé-Perthes.

NATURAL HISTORY

The natural history of Legg-Calvé-Perthes disease has been difficult to study accurately because treatment programs were undertaken as soon as the disease was recognized. Legg's five patients were all treated in some manner; one was even treated surgically. Thus, there are really no pure natural history studies of completely untreated patients, and it has been necessary to infer the probable natural history by studying groups of patients treated with means now considered ineffective. This involves accepting the assumption that these often rigorous programs of nonweight-bearing, cast immobilization, and use of Patten bottom braces had no effect, either favorable or adverse, on the course of the disease. For example, in an often quoted "natural history" study by Gower and Johnston,[118] two patients suffered growth arrests from epiphyseal compression in spica casts that were not changed for upwards of 4 months. Although it is unlikely that treatment in a spica cast for up to 23 months had no effect on the outcome of the hip, to gain some understanding of the disease process, these studies must be accepted, albeit with reservations, because other resources are not available. These and other studies have indicated that the disease is an extremely variable disorder (Cases 1-6; Figures 17-22). Some children have minimal symptoms and little change in their femoral head over the course of the disease. However, the majority have moderate symptoms and a difficult 12 to 18 months followed by resolution of symptoms and return to full activity. A few children have severe symptoms throughout the course of the disorder and remain symptomatic into early adulthood.

The most consistent and frequently documented factor in outcome is the age at onset.[119-124] Younger children, especially those with onset before 6 years of age, tend to have a mild course and good outcome, except for a few cases that do poorly. Children between 6 and 9 years old at onset have moderate symptoms, with a few more doing poorly but the majority still doing well. Children 9 years old and older have a higher frequency of poor results and a more difficult course of disease overall.

Radiographic involvement is also variable, and many classification schemes have been used to assess severity. Legg[7] recognized two types, the "cap" and the "mushroom" types with the mushroom type being less common but more severe. Waldenström[95] noted three types, with the most severe being less common. Catterall[124] proposed a four-part classification augmented by risk factors that when present increased the likelihood of a poor outcome. The Lateral Pillar classification proposed by this author grades involvement of the lateral portion of the femoral head into groups A, B, and C.[96] These systems, which are discussed in more detail below, all correlate more or less with final outcome, with the worst results coming from the most severely involved hips.

Duration of disease also correlates with outcome, and those with the greatest delay in healing have the poorest outcome. In the Herring and associates[96] series, hips classified as lateral pillar group C hips healed in 67 months compared to group A hips with healing in 37 months and group B in 50 months. The outcome was 100% good/excellent in group A, 79% good/excellent in group B, and 29% good/excellent in group C.

CLASSIFICATION

The clinical course and final outcome in Legg-Calvé-Perthes disease vary considerably between different patients, and many attempts have been made to classify the radiographic findings in a way that correlates with the severity of the disease. Legg[7] described two types that he called the cap type and the mushroom type, the former implying a flattened femoral head and the latter a round or oval shape. Waldenström[95] described three types, the first two associated with a good outcome and the third with a poor result. He should be considered the father of several "risk signs" because he notes that lateralization of the femoral head and metaphyseal lucencies suggest a poor prognosis. He noted that the final result in type three hips is a conical shape of both the femoral head and the acetabulum that reduces the range of motion to the plane of flexion and extension. Goff[1] described three types also, a spherical type, a cap type, and an irregular type.

CASE STUDIES

The six sets of illustrations in this section illustrate the varying courses taken by Legg-Calvé-Perthes disease and, in themselves, represent a succinct atlas of the disease. In these examples, the course of the disease and the final outcome vary with the age of the child at onset. Children younger than 5 years of age at onset tend to have a milder course of the disease and a better outcome than older children.

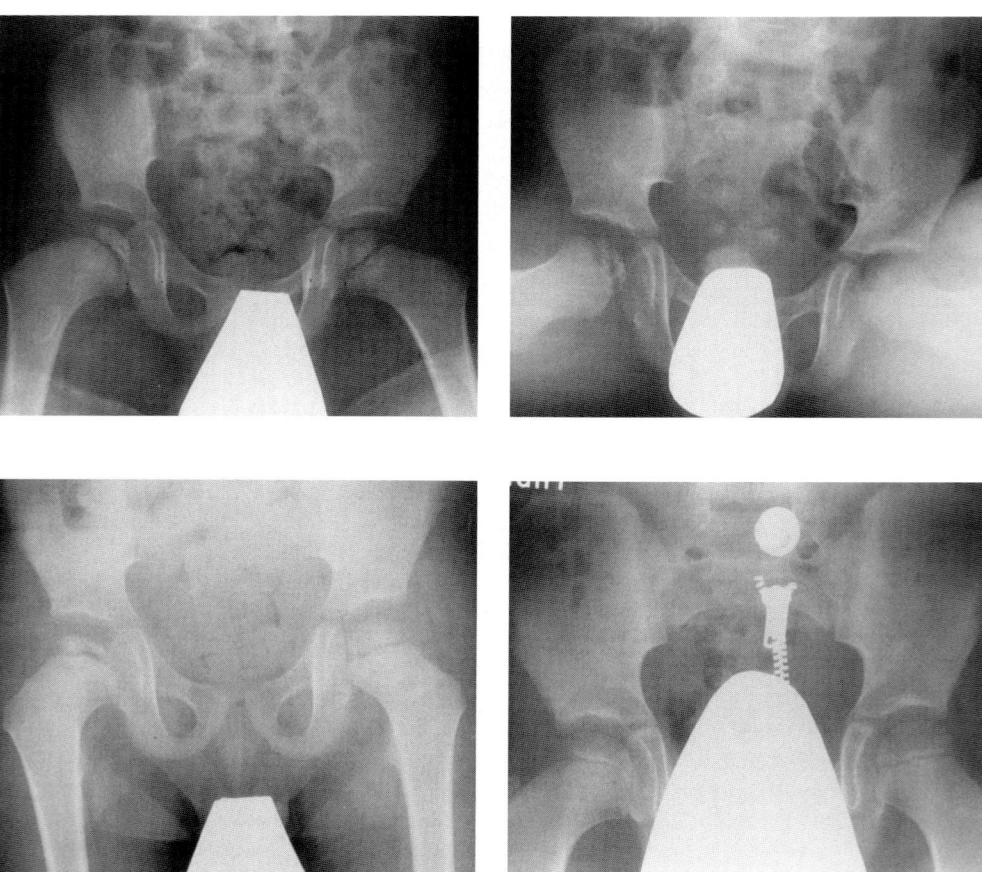

FIGURE 17

Case I. This young child had a very mild course as often is seen in children younger than 5 years old at onset. He was 3 years 1 month old and had a slight limp when first seen by the physician. **Top left,** Anteroposterior (AP) radiograph at the time of onset showing increased density within a smaller femoral head. A small crescent of lucency hearalds the onset of the fragmentation stage. **Top right,** Frog lateral radiograph at presentation showing uniform involvement in the femoral head. **Bottom left,** AP radiograph 1 month after onset showing a smaller femoral head on the right with increased density laterally and loss of height in the medial and middle portions of the head. This is classified as a lateral pillar group B because there is some loss of height in the lateral pillar. **Bottom right,** AP radiograph 5 years after onset. The femoral head is round with an essentially normal contour. This will go on to a Stulberg group I or II classification and a Mose good.

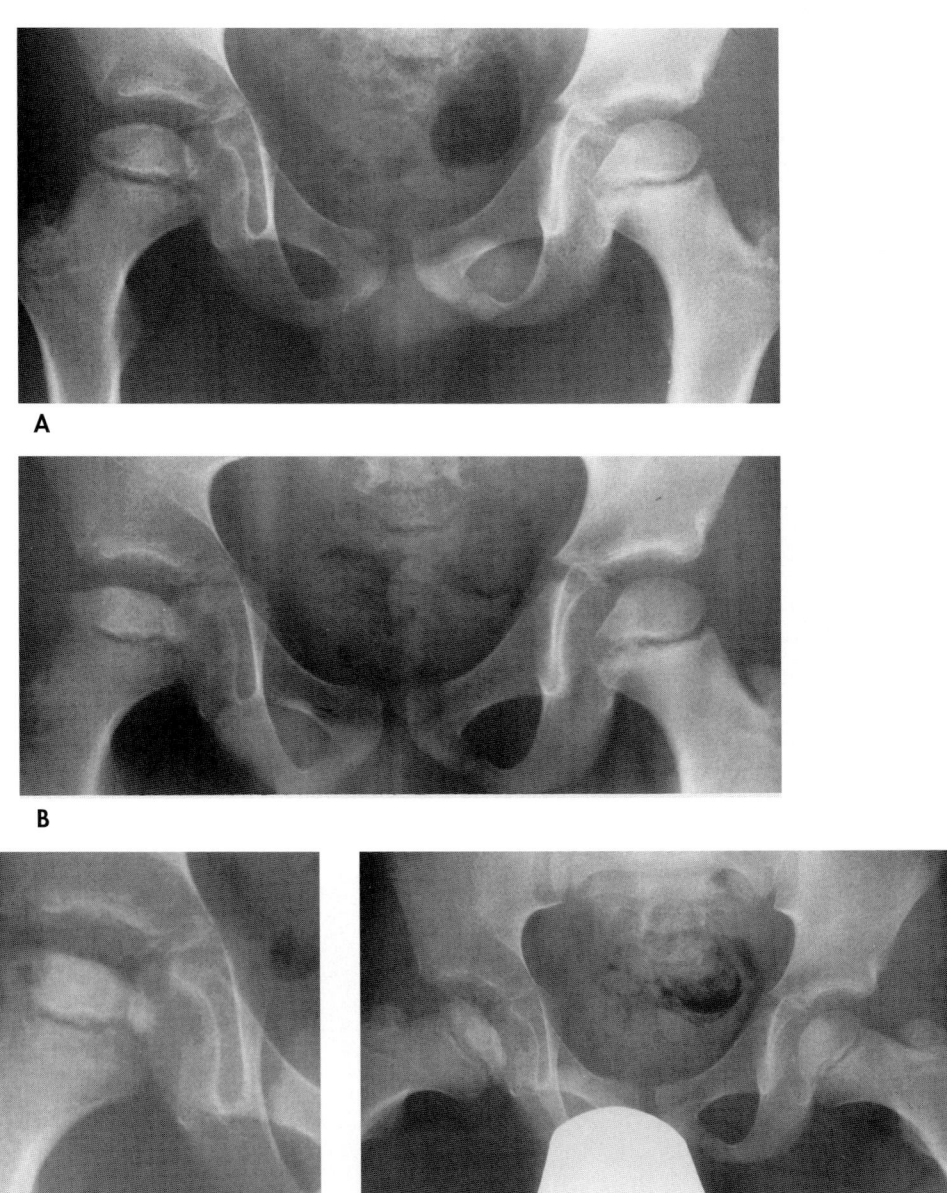

FIGURE 18

Case 2. A boy 6 years 10 months of age at onset of Legg-Calvé-Perthes disease. His course of disease is fairly typical for this age, one of moderate symptoms resolving over 12 months. The lateral pillar classification is group B. He was treated with an orthosis. Six years after onset he had new symptoms related to an osteochondral fragment. **A,** Initial radiograph. There is slight increased density of the femoral head and some widening of the distance from the head to the medial teardrop figure. **B,** Anteroposterior (AP) radiograph 1 month later showing further increased density centrally within the femoral head. The hip is in the stage of increased density. At this point the hip would be classified as a lateral pillar B. **C,** AP radiograph 4 months after onset. There is now a demarcation between the central portion of the femoral head and the lateral and medial segments. The lucency in the lateral portion suggests that the onset of fragmentation will occur soon. **D,** Abduction-internal rotation radiograph 5 months after onset. The femoral head seats well into the acetabulum. *(Continued on next page.)*

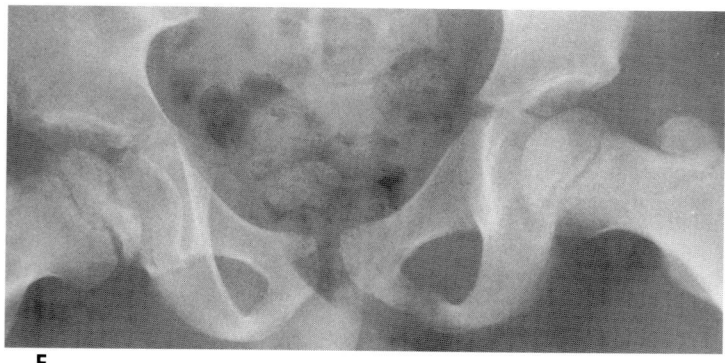

E

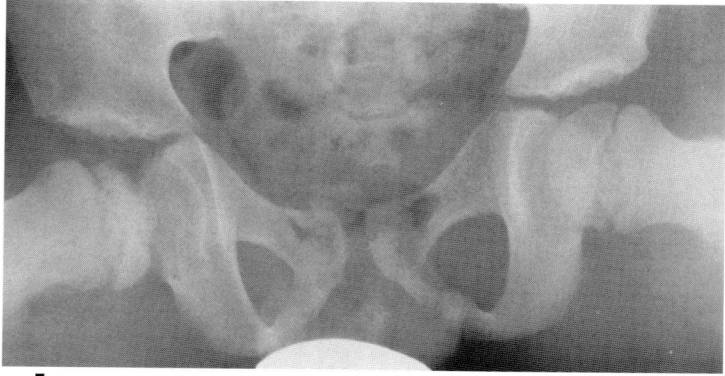

F

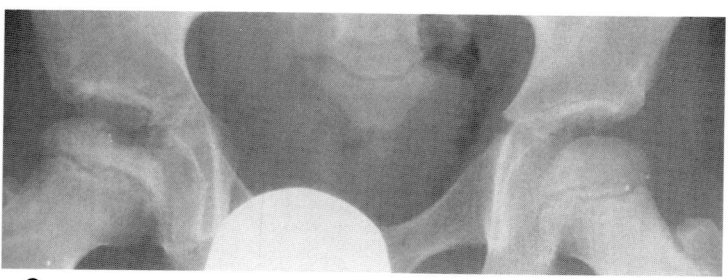

G

FIGURE 18 (CONTINUED FROM PREVIOUS PAGE.)

Case 2. A boy 6 years 10 months of age at onset of Legg-Calvé-Perthes disease. His course of disease is fairly typical for this age, one of moderate symptoms resolving over 12 months. The lateral pillar classification is group B. He was treated with an orthosis. Six years after onset he had new symptoms related to an osteochondral fragment. **E,** Anteroposterior (AP) radiograph 10 months after onset. The femoral head is reaching the stage of reossification after an abreviated fragmentation stage. The contour of the head is preserved. **F,** Frog lateral radiograph 10 months after onset. New bone formation may be seen in the subchondral areas of the head. **G,** AP radiograph 15 months after onset. There is further healing of the avascular necrosis and the contour of the head is improving.

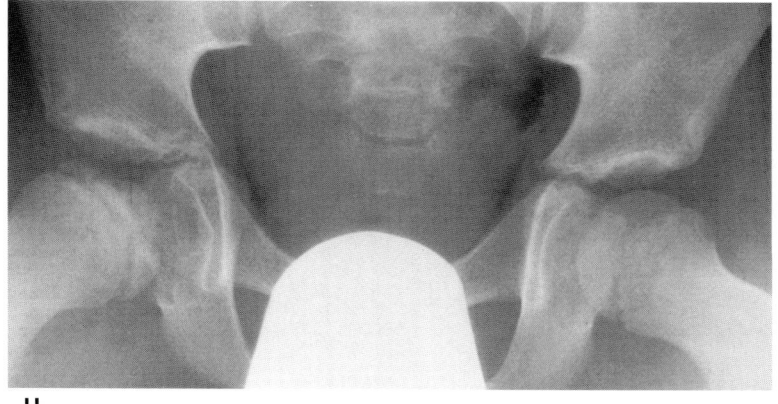

H

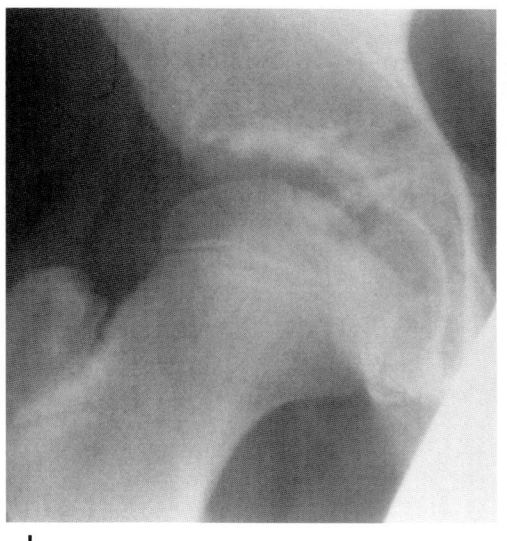

I

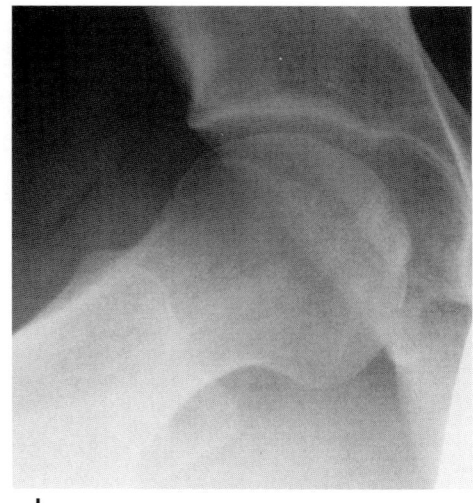

J

FIGURE 18 (CONTINUED FROM PREVIOUS PAGE.)
H, Frog lateral radiograph shows further addition of new bone. **I,** Anteroposterior radiograph 6 years 2 months after onset. The head has a round contour but there is a central fragment that appears to be separate from the head. **J,** Frog lateral radiograph showing the central fragment that is undisplaced. The patient had occasional mechanical symptoms but was generally doing well and no treatment was instituted.

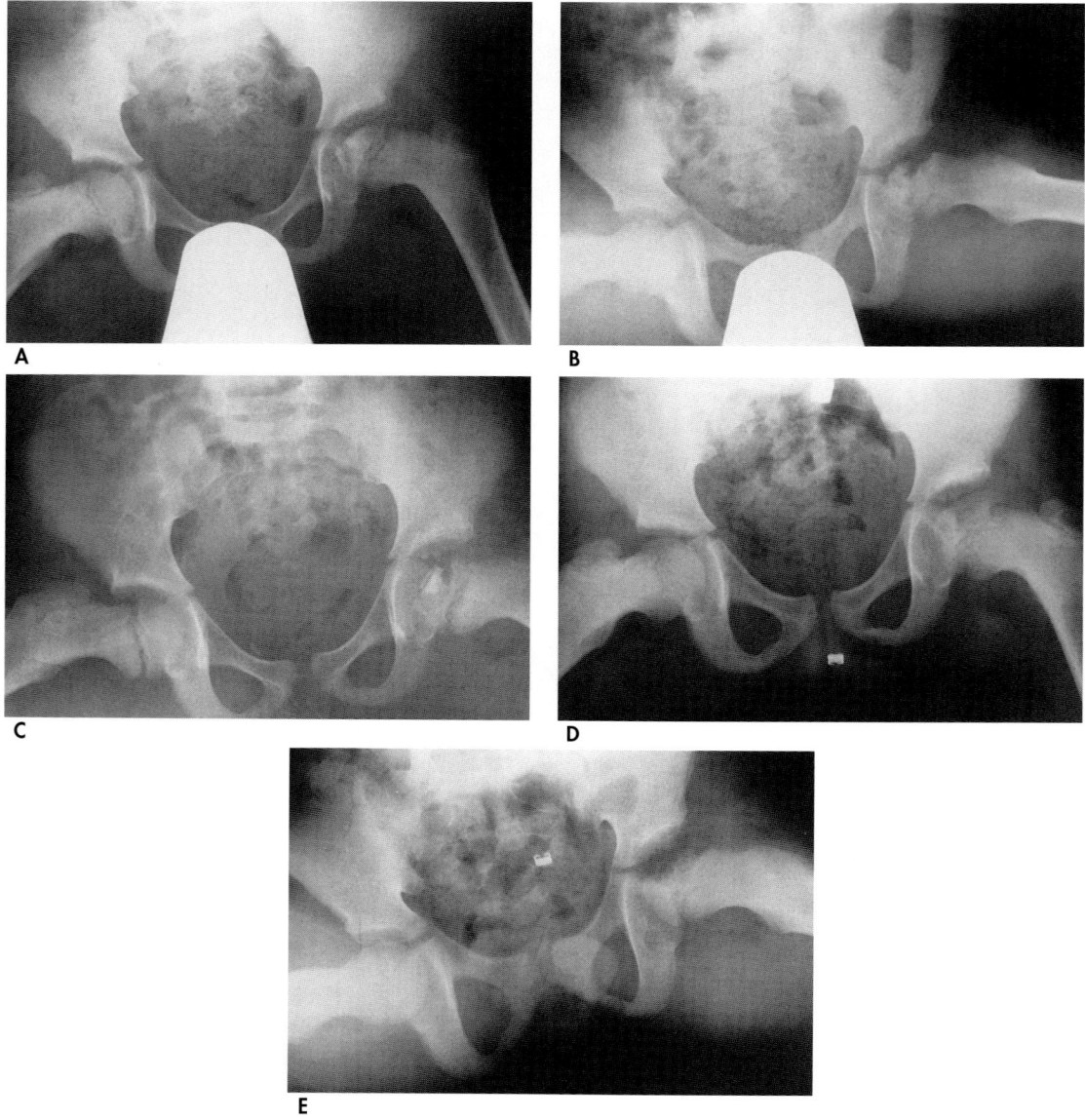

FIGURE 19

Case 3. A boy with onset of Legg-Calve-Perthes at age 7 years 1 month. His course of disease is prolonged with a poor outcome. This is an uncommon sequence of events that may defy treatment efforts. **A,** Initial anteroposterior (AP) radiograph showing increased radiodensity in the central portion of the femoral head. The central lucency in the head suggests that the fragmentation stage is about to begin. **B,** Initial frog lateral radiograph showing involvement anteriorly and centrally. **C,** AP radiograph several months later showing further fragmentation. The lateral pillar can now be visualized and is just about half the height of the contralateral femoral head. This would be classified as a lateral pillar B (but almost a C), **D,** AP radiograph 1 year after onset. The femoral head is well into the healing phase and the contour is slightly flattened. **E,** Frog lateral radiograph 1 year after onset showing persistent lucency anteriorly. **F,** Anteroposterior (AP) radiograph 7 years after onset. The contour of the head is almost round and healing appears complete. **G,** Frog lateral radiograph 7 years after onset shows that there is an anterior portion of the head that has not reossified. The femoral head contour is much less round on this projection. **H,** An arthrogram 7 years after onset shows a round surface to the femoral head. **I,** A tomogram 7 years after onset shows a large unossified fragment in the anterior central portion of the femoral head. A portion of the loose fragment was removed but the symptoms were not relieved. **J,** Anteroposterior radiograph 9 years after onset showing some flattening of the femoral head. **K,** A frog lateral radiograph 9 years after onset showing persistent lucent area with incomplete reossification.

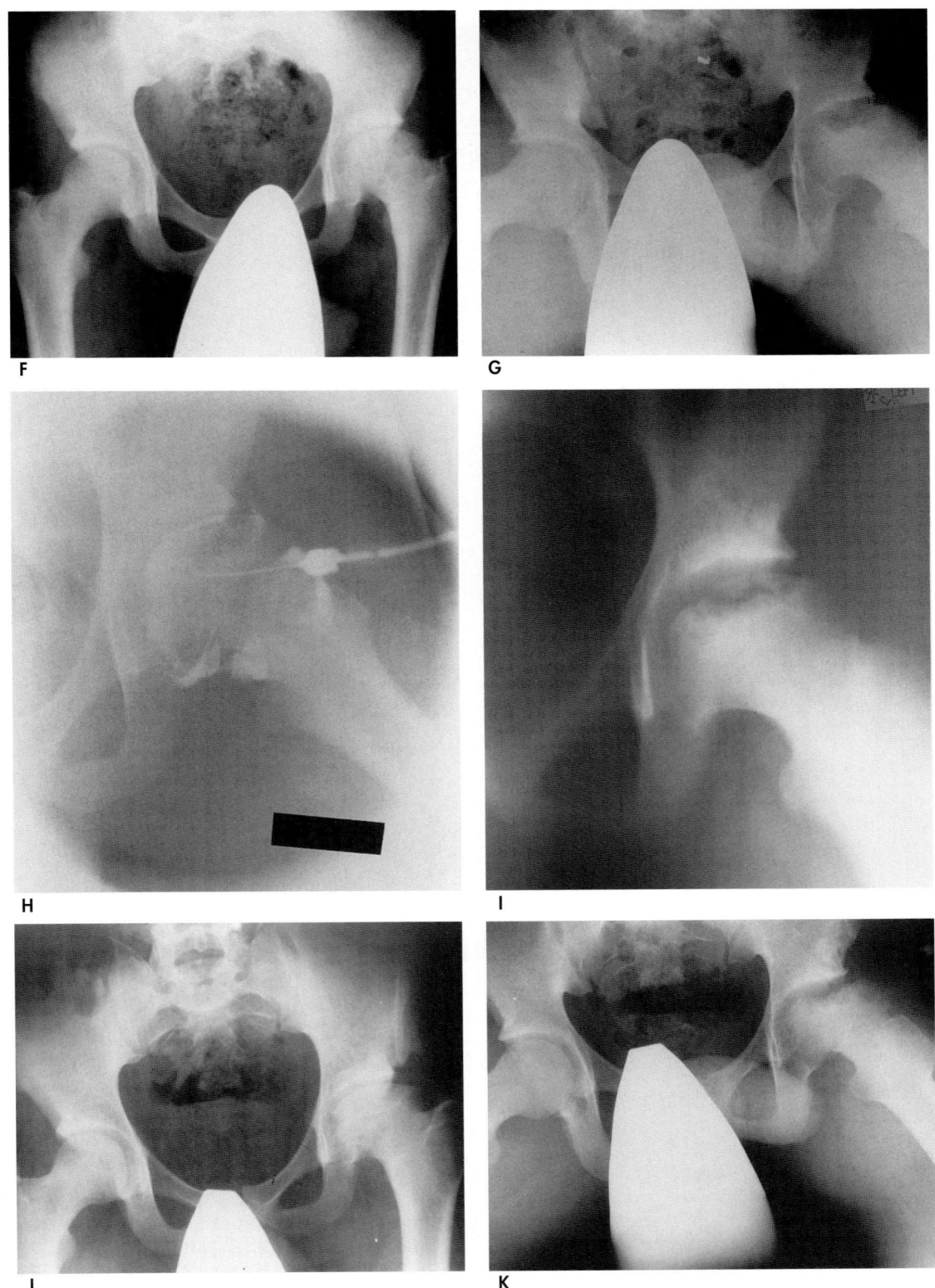

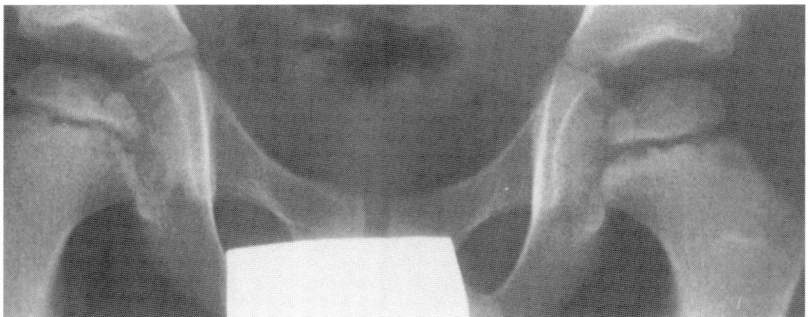

A

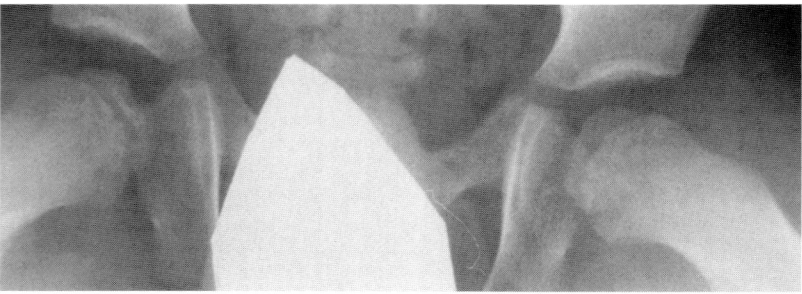

B

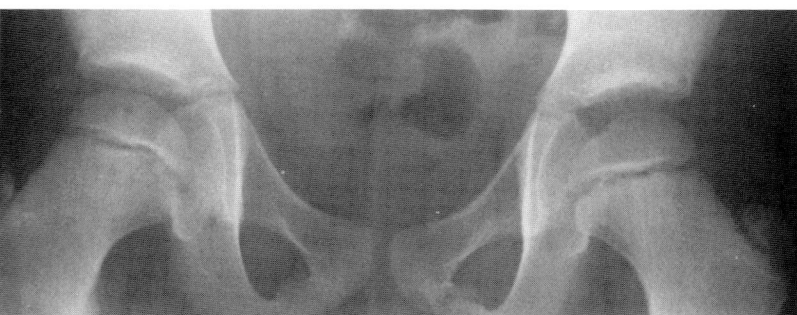

C

FIGURE 20
Case 4. A 4 year 9 month old boy with recent onset of a limp. Minimal changes involve only the central portion of the femoral head. The radiographic changes gradually evolve and resemble Legg-Calvé-Perthes but may be some other process. These changes are seen at times in the contralateral hip of a patient with more typical Legg Perthes. **A,** Anteroposterior (AP) radiograph showing lucencies within the right femoral head, which is smaller than the contralateral femoral head. This would be classified as lateral pillar group A. **B,** Frog lateral radiograph showing central areas of radiolucency in the right femoral head. **C,** AP radiograph 3 years after onset of symptoms showing almost complete resolution of the changes in the femoral head.

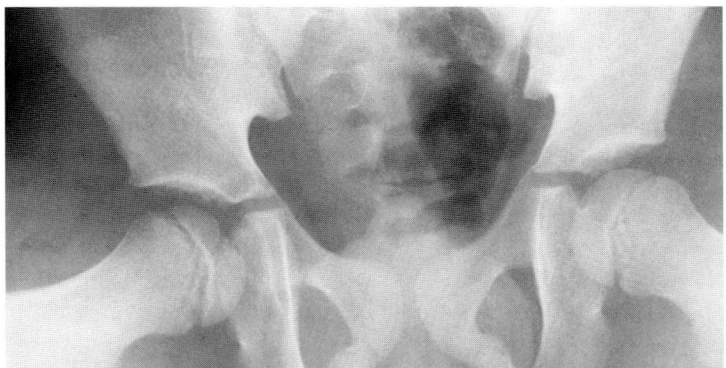

D

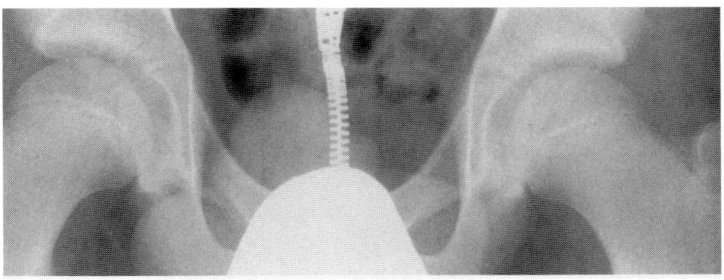

E

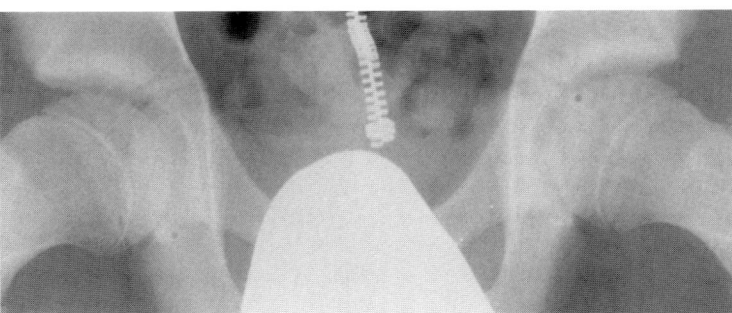

F

D, Frog lateral radiograph 3 years after onset demonstrating a residual central lucency in the femoral head. **E,** AP radiograph 9 years after onset. The femoral head now appears normal with no evidence of the prior lesion. **F,** Frog lateral radiograph 9 years after onset with no change in femoral head contour. This hip is classified as a Stulberg I result, not distinguishable from normal.

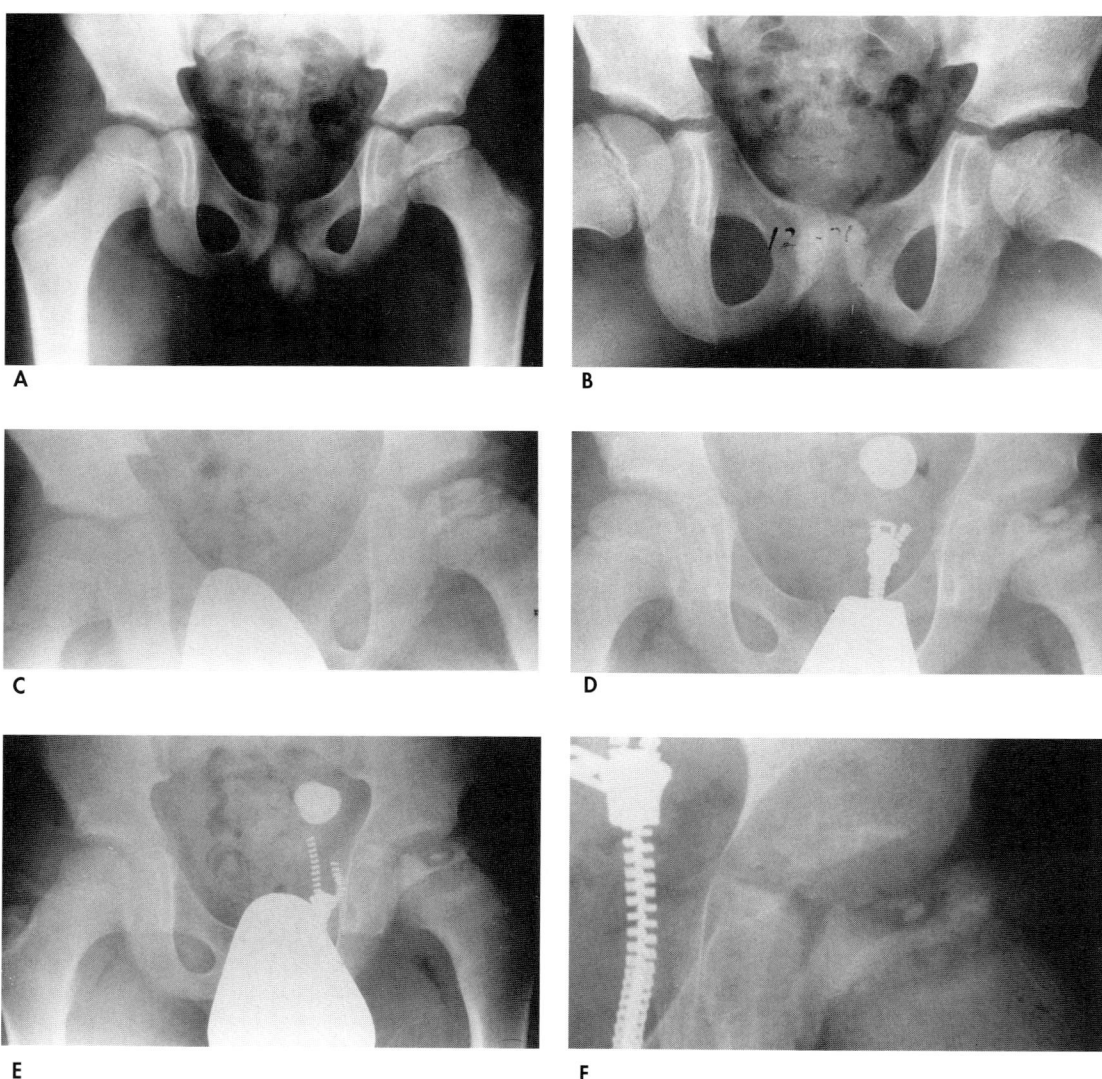

FIGURE 21

Case 5. A 10-year 11-month old boy with recent onset of hip pain. The femoral head gradually improves its shape over time. This is a manifestation of a benign natural history rather than response to treatment because these changes occur over many years after brace treatment was stopped. **A,** Anteroposterior (AP) radiograph at the time of onset. There is slight increase in the radiodensity of the femoral head and mild widening of the joint space. **B,** Initial frog lateral radiograph showing a radiolucent crescent over the anterior two fifths of the femoral head. **C,** AP radiograph 9 months after onset. The central fragment has separated from the lateral pillar and has collapsed relative to the lateral pillar. There is lucency in the lateral pillar but minimal collapse; this is a good example of a lateral pillar B. There is considerable extrusion of the femoral head. **D,** AP radiograph 13 months after onset. There is new bone formation in the lateral pillar area signaling the beginning of the reossification stage. Brace treatment was stopped at this time. **E,** Anteroposterior (AP) radiograph 17 months after onset showing further reossification laterally. There is still marked extrusion of the femoral head. **F,** AP radiograph 22 months after onset. Note the bicompartmental shape of the acetabulum. **G,** AP radiograph 4 years after onset. The femoral head is flattened and the acetabulum is still irregular. **H,** Frog lateral 4 years after onset. The femoral head is almost round. **I,** Anteroposterior radiograph almost 6 years after onset. The femoral head has continued to become rounder and is better seated within the acetabulum. **J,** Frog lateral radiograph showing further rounding up of the femoral head. Because of the oval shape of the femoral head on this view this hip would be classified as c Stulberg III result. Many such hips continue to improve and become Stulberg II results.

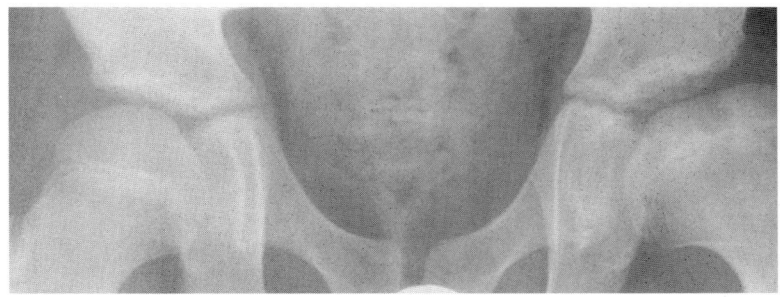

G

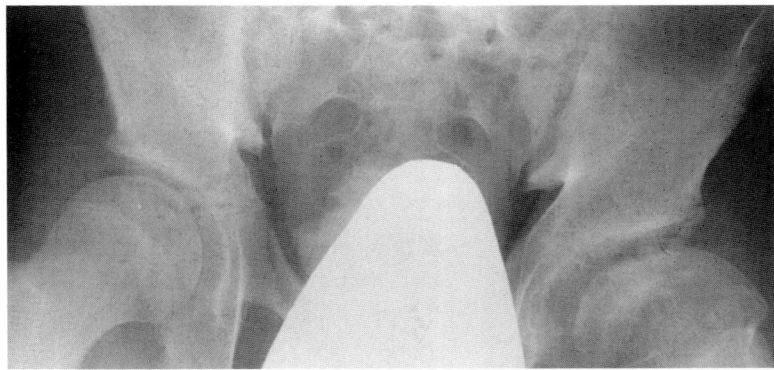

H

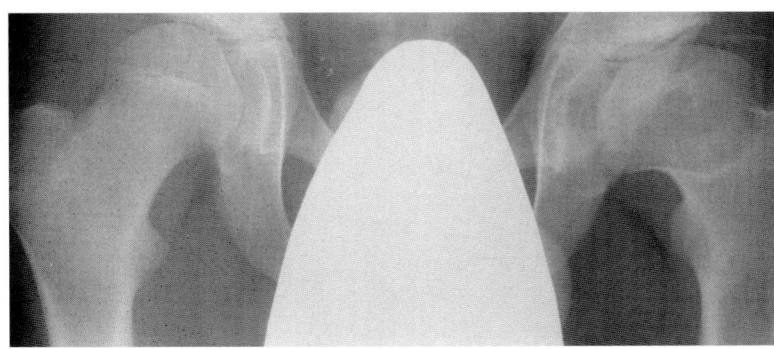

I

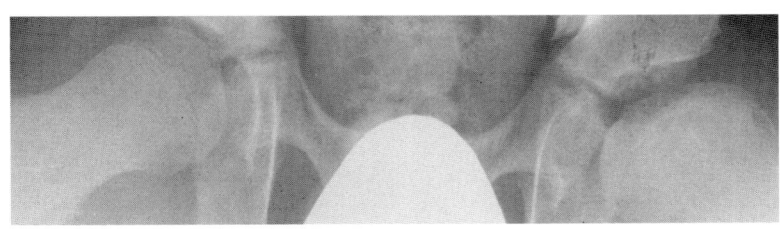

J

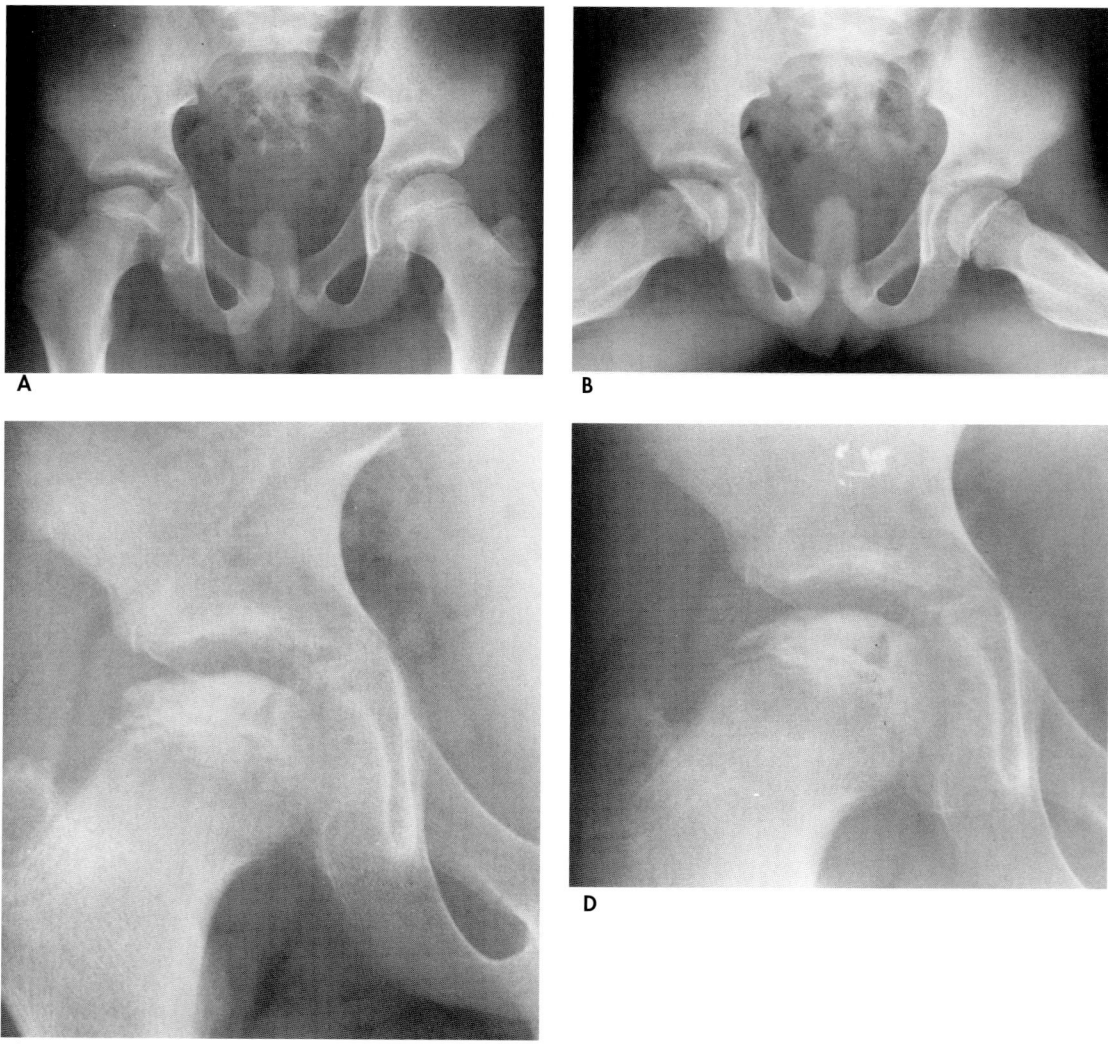

FIGURE 22

Case 6. A 10-year 10-month old boy with symptoms for one month. The changes evolve over a long period of time and result in femoral head deformity. This course is typical of patients whose onset is over age 10 years. This is a lateral pillar type C. **A,** Anteroposterior (AP) radiograph showing increased density of the femoral head with widening of the joint space. **B,** A frog lateral radiograph showing a small subchondral fracture anteriorly. In my experience, the extent of the subchondral fracture does not predict subsequent head involvement. **C,** AP radiograph 10 months later. The head remains in the stage of increased density. The lateral pillar is depressed along with the central segment. **D,** AP radiograph 1 year after onset. Lucencies in the lateral pillar and centrally indicate the start of the fragmentation stage. At this point the lateral pillar is depressed more than the central portion and more than half its original height. This would be a lateral pillar C classification. **E,** AP radiograph 14 months after onset. The lateral pillar is almost completely lucent while the central density remains. **F,** An arthrogram 17 months after onset showing flattening of the femoral head and acetabulum. With abduction there is pooling of dye in the acetabulum. **G,** AP radiograph 2 years after onset. The healing phase has begun as evidenced by new bone formation in the lateral pillar. The femoral head has an ovoid shape. **H,** AP radiograph 26 months after onset showing further reossification of the entire femoral head. **I,** AP radiograph 4 years 5 months after onset. The femoral head is fully reossified and the head is flattened. **J,** Frog lateral radiograph 4 years 5 months after onset. There is flattening of the femoral head on this view also. This hip is a Stulberg IV result.

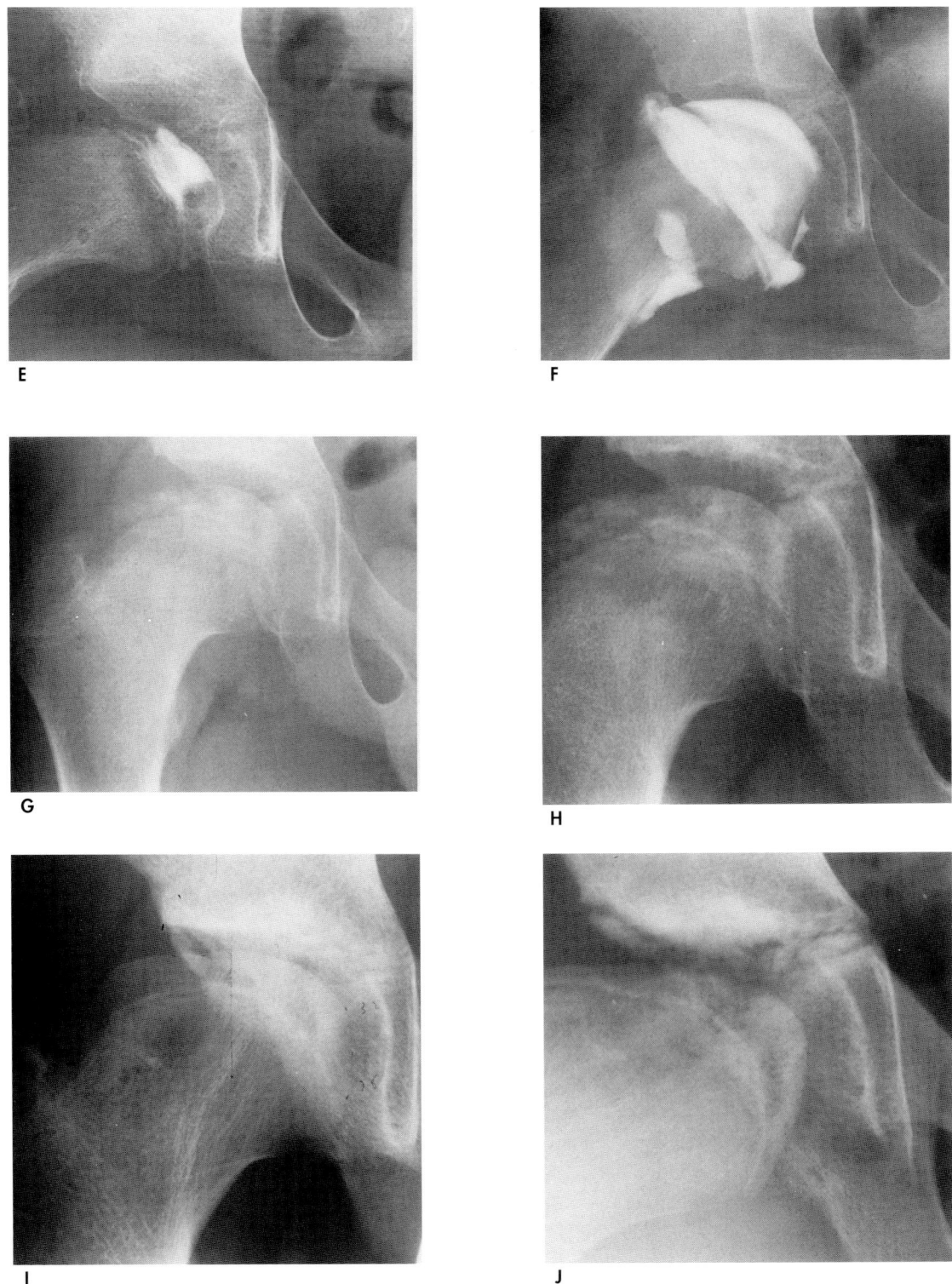

E

F

G

H

I

J

Catterall The introduction of the Catterall classification in 1971 was an important event in the evolution of the care of Legg-Calvé-Perthes disease. At the time of its publication, most centers used very vigorous treatment programs for all patients.[124] Catterall proposed four groups and stated that groups I and II had a benign prognosis and did not require treatment, whereas groups III and IV should be treated (Fig. 23). He also proposed a group of "head at risk" factors that foretold a poor prognosis. The groups were described in general terms, and subsequent studies have shown that different observers are unable to reproduce the classification when given test radiographs.[125,126] Nonetheless, Catterall's work initiated the search for reliable prognostic indicators and emphasized the concept that many patients will fare well without any intervention. (Both Legg[14] and Waldenström[15] pointed out the fact that many patients did well without treatment, but their insight was forgotten over the years.)

In Catterall's group I, only the anterior part of the epiphysis is involved. In group II, there is formation of a central sequestrum with more of the anterior segment involved. The involved segment may collapse, but the epiphyseal height is maintained. In group III, only a small part of the epiphysis is not "sequestrated" (Catterall's term) with the uninvolved parts lying medially and laterally to the central segment. In group IV, the entire epiphysis is sequestrated. The "head at risk" was defined as having four possible risk signs, Gage's sign of a radiolucent "v" in the lateral portion of the epiphysis, calcification lateral to the epiphysis, lateral subluxation of the femoral head, and a horizontal physeal line.

Christensen and associates[126] studied the ability of four experienced observers to apply the Catterall classification and found a low and, in their opinion, unacceptable degree of interobserver agreement even when groups II and III were combined. Hardcastle and associates[125] found a similar lack of reproducibility, especially in delineating groups I, II, and III, with better performance with group IV and when groups II and III were combined.

Interpretation of risk signs was also unsatisfactory.[125] Van Dam and associates[127] found that Catterall classification was changed in 40% of hips if applied before fragmentation, and only in 6% if applied during the fragmentation stage. (This is not surprising because Catterall based the classification on radiographs during the fragmentation stage.)

Risk Factors A number of authors have studied the prognostic significance of various risk factors (Figs. 18, *C,* and 21, *D* and *E*). Dickens and Menelaus[128] found four reliable prognostic factors: the extent of uncovering of the femoral head, the Catterall classification, lateral calcification, and lateral head displacement using the head to teardrop distance. Poussa and associates[129] also noted four factors associated with a poor prognosis: lateral calcification, widening of the femoral head before fragmentation, the saturn phenomenon (a sclerotic epiphysis surrounded by a ring of lucency), and widening of the femoral neck in the early phases of disease. Mukherjee and Fabry[130] found that the only head at risk factor with prognostic significance was lateralization of the femoral head, and they found no correlation with outcome of metaphyseal reaction, Gage's sign, lateral calcification, and a horizontal growth plate. Yrjonen and associates[131] found that lateral calcification was a very poor prognostic sign, as was widening of the epiphysis in the early fragmentation stage or before. They noted that bicompartmentalization of the acetabulum was also not a useful prognosticator.

Lateral Pillar The lateral pillar classification proposed by Herring and associates[96] consists of three groups. This classification is based on the radiographic changes seen in the lateral segment of the femoral head on the AP radiograph. This concept was first noted by Ferguson[132] who stated that if the lateral segment is present, it becomes the weightbearing strut to guard the central avascular segment from harm.[11] When this separation is present, the central fragment will be depressed relative to the lateral pillar.[133]

The lateral pillar classification can be determined from AP radiographs as the femoral head enters the fragmentation stage (Fig. 19). At the onset of fragmentation, there often is spontaneous demarcation between the central, medial, and lateral portions (or pillars) of the femoral head. In group A, there is little density change in the lateral portion of the head and no loss of height of that segment (Fig. 20). In group B, there is lucency and subsequent loss of height in the lateral pillar that does not exceed 50% of the original height as judged by the contralateral hip or

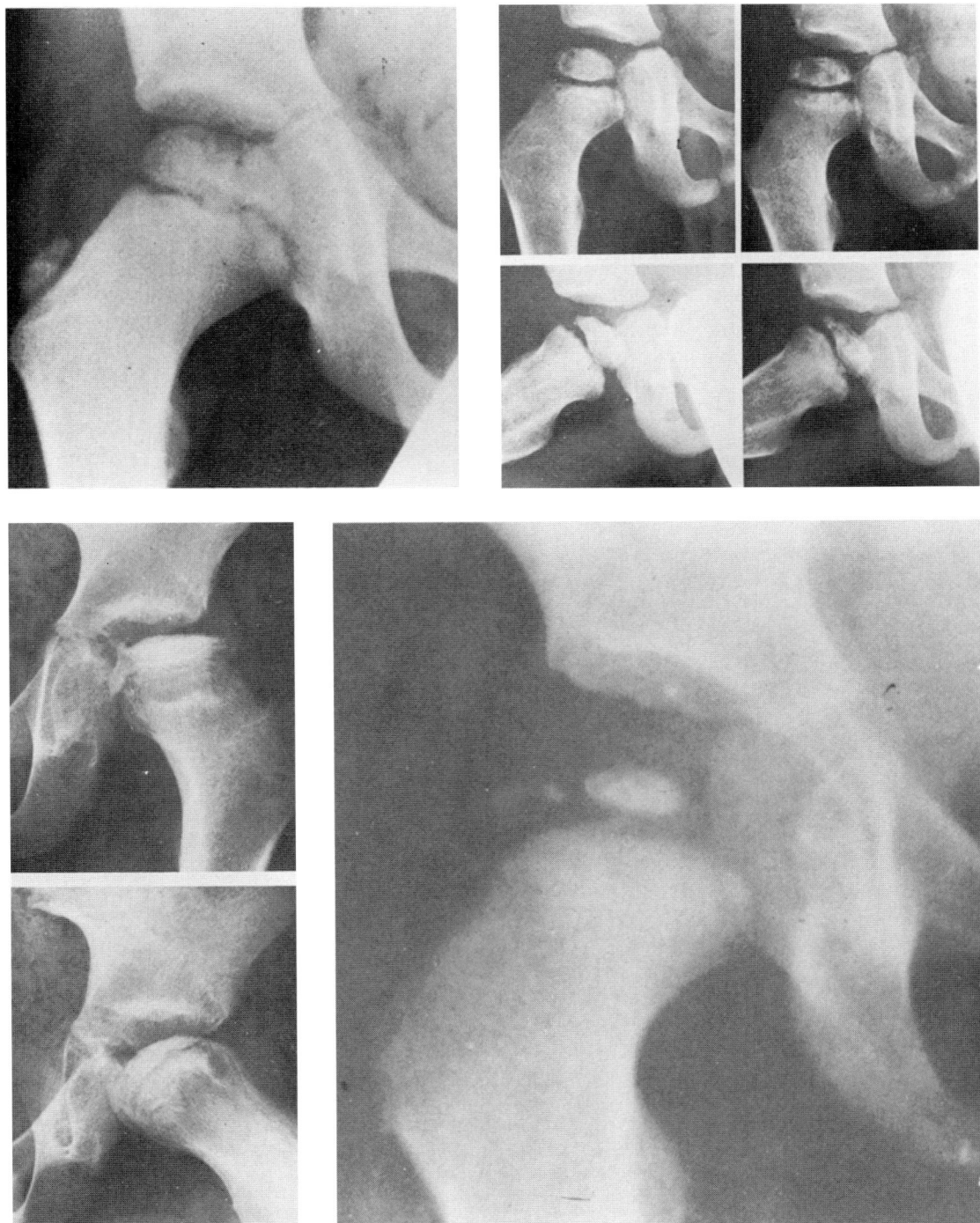

FIGURE 23

Catterall's original figures showing his classification. **Top left,** A group I case. **Top right,** A group II case. **Bottom left,** A group III case. **Bottom right,** A group IV case. (Reproduced with permission from Catterall A, Pringle J, Byers PD, et al: A review of the morphology of Perthes' disease. *J Bone Joint Surg* 1982;64B:269-275.)

by earlier radiographs. An early sign of group B behavior is collapse of the central fragment beneath the level of the lateral pillar (Fig. 21). As fragmentation evolves, the lateral pillar may lose height and may extrude laterally, but should not collapse beyond half its original height. In group C, there is early lucency in the lateral pillar and little or no demarcation between the lateral and central segments, with subsequent collapse of the lateral pillar to less than 50% of its original height (Fig. 22). The lateral segment often is lower in height than the central segment quite early in the fragmentation stage. Subsequent studies have shown a strong correlation between the lateral pillar classification and the eventual outcome of the hip.[96]

The experimental work of Rab and associates[133] suggests a mechanical basis for a good result when the lateral pillar is preserved. They performed a finite element analysis of femoral head stresses and found that if only the central portion of the femoral head was necrotic, the remaining lateral rim of bone would stress shield the central core and prevent collapse. When there was extensive necrosis, the shielding effect was lost and the head collapsed. Ritterbusch and associates[134] compared the interobserver reliability of the Catterall and lateral pillar classifications. They found that the lateral pillar classification was more predictive of the final outcome of the hip and that the interobserver reliability was greater than that of the Catterall classification.

Mose In addition to the classifications proposed for severity, several end result classifications have been in common use. Because femoral head changes occur with growth, these classifications should be applied to the skeletally mature femoral head (Figs. 21 and 24). Mose[135] proposed matching the shape of the healed femoral head to a template of concentric circles. A good result by the Mose criteria is one in which the femoral head contour deviates no more than 1 mm from a given circle on both the AP and frog lateral radiographs. In a fair result, the contour of the femoral head must fall within 2 mm of a circle on both radiographic views, and in a poor result, the femoral head deviates from a circle by more than 2 mm. Mose's actual statement about the classification is confusing; he stated, "To be classified spherical, the surface of the head must follow the same circle on the template within a variation of

2 mm or 1 mm both in frontal and lateral views."[135] This classification is easily reproduced, but is a very strict one that does not describe the many different possible results.

Stulberg Stulberg and associates[136] proposed a reproducible five-part classification of end results. In group I, the contour of the hip is essentially normal (Fig. 20, E). In group II, there is some loss of height of the femoral head, but the contour of the head matches a concentric circle within 2 mm on both the AP and frog lateral radiographs (Fig. 18, I and J). Group III hips are more elliptically shaped, and the head deviates from a circle by more than 2 mm (Fig. 21, I and J). In group IV, there is true flattening of the femoral head (Fig. 22, I and J). (Unfortunately, Stulberg and associates[136] fail to define how great a segment of the head must be flat to qualify as a group IV.) In groups III and IV the femoral head and acetabulum are of the same shape, and they call this "congruous incongruity." Group V hips are those in older patients in which there is collapse of the femoral head without corresponding changes in the acetabulum. These resemble adult osteonecrosis with central head collapse, and are termed "incongruous incongruity." The studies by Stulberg and associates[136] showed that subsequent arthritic changes were well predicted by the classification.

OUTCOME

The long-term prognosis is directly related to the shape of the healed femoral head. The authors who have assessed long-term outcome have reported variable rates of late degenerative arthritis, but there is general agreement that head shape is the most important predictor of future prognosis.[118,137]

The early studies of natural history had very optimistic results, whereas later studies with longer follow-up have shown increasing rates of late degenerative arthritis. Eaton[138] reported on 100 hips in 88 patients followed up for an average of 19 years (range: 10 to 43 years). He found 64% good or excellent, 17% fair, and 19% poor results. Three hips had arthrodesis. Sixty-three patients had no limp, eight limped after excessive activity, and 14 had a constant limp. Seven had less than 50% of normal motion and seven had enough pain to consider surgery. Treatment for most of these patients was bed rest with or without traction. An interesting finding was that 13 of

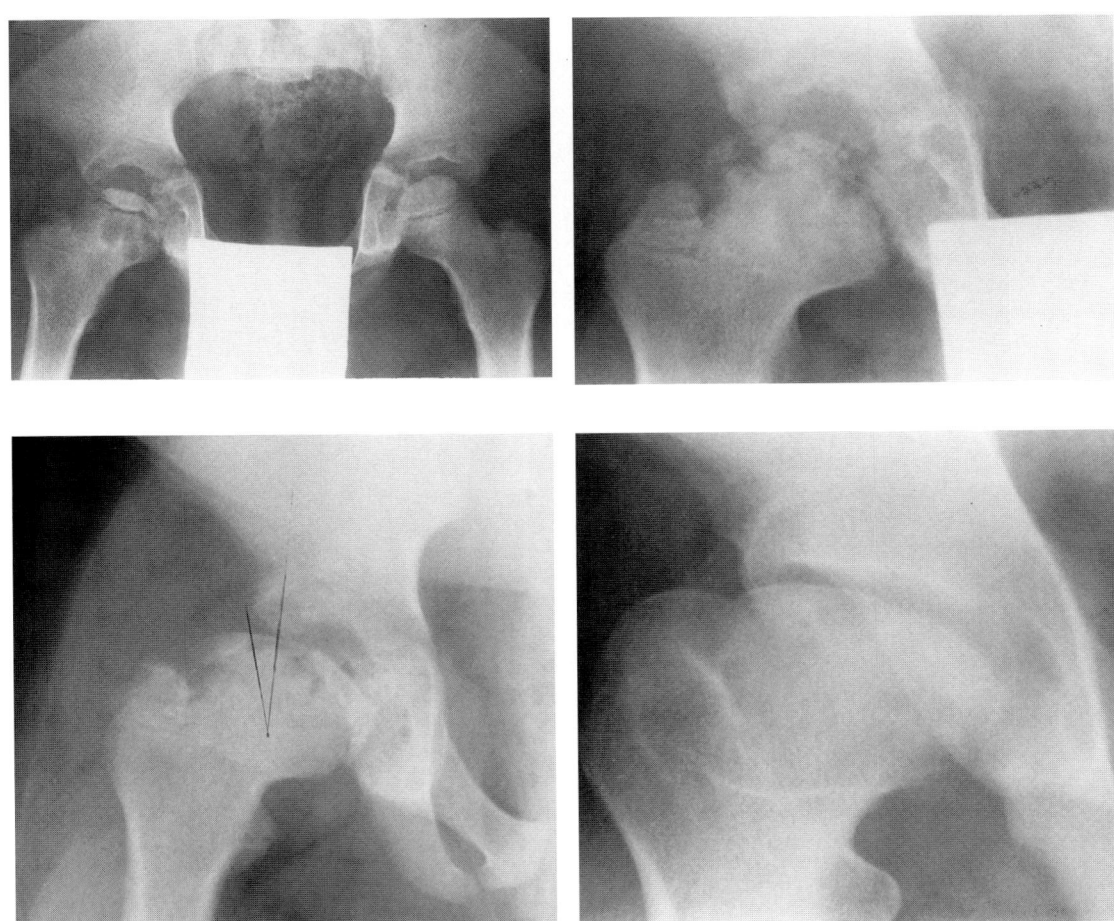

FIGURE 24
A 4-year 8-month old boy with intermittent symptoms for 6 months. Although a benign course would be expected in this age group, the reossification period in this child is prolonged over 4 years, during which the head progressively flattens. **Top left,** Anteroposterior (AP) radiograph at onset showing a central dense segment, widening of the joint space, and metaphyseal lucency. **Top right,** AP radiograph 15 months after onset. Reossification has begun in the lateral pillar. The joint space remains widened. **Bottom left,** AP radiograph 3.5 years after onset. The femoral head is ovoid and reossification is incomplete centrally. **Bottom right,** AP radiograph 11 years after onset. The head is fully reossified and is ovoid, a Stulberg group III result.

16 patients untreated or treated with less than 6 months of bed rest had good or excellent results.

Ratliff[139] reported 34 hips observed for an average of 30 years (range: 25 to 40 years). Treatment in 25 was immobilization on frames for an average of 18 months (range: 6 to 24 months). Eight were untreated. Fifteen had good, 11 fair, and eight poor results. Thirty had no pain, and 29 did normal activities. No change was noted from 1953 to 1965 in some patients. Four out of five were fully active and pain free, but only two of five had good radiographic findings.

Out of 112 patients initially treated, Gower and Johnston[118] contacted 66 patients and had 36 return for follow-up. The age at examination was 44.6 years (range: 30 to 48 years) with follow-up of an average of 36.3 years. Average age at onset of symptoms was 8.3 years. Treatment in 28 had been spica cast for 1 to 23 months. Two had growth arrests of either distal femur or proximal tibia from lack of spica cast change. Thirteen had no pain, seven had pain after work, eight limited their walking for pain, and two had pain after a few hours work or a few blocks walking. Range of motion was good except for six with a flexion contracture. Thirty had round heads; 22, flattened; and two, angular heads, and there were 17 normal, 12 narrowed, and one absent joint space. Seven had no degenerative changes, 16 had minimal changes, six had moderate changes, and one had severe degenerative changes. The Iowa hip score was a mean of 91 out of 100. Seven patients over 50 years old averaged 90 on the Iowa scale. Age at onset had little effect on outcome. Only three patients had surgery for hip problems.[118]

Englehardt[140] followed up 55 patients for 42 years and found disabling arthritis in only nine hips; 46% had excellent and 33% good late results. Lateral calcification, age at onset, and loss of sphericity of the head were correlated with late degenerative problems. Englehardt[140] did not find a correlation between the Catterall classification and outcome. Saito and associates[141] studied 56 hips with average follow-up of 18 years and found 13 with coxarthrosis. Steepness of the lateral edge of the acetabulum was the most significant prognostic factor leading to degenerative disease. Perpich and associates[142] reviewed 40 adults at an average of 30 years following treatment with spica casts. He found 85% had good results, 5% fair, and 10% poor results. Better results were correlated with diagnosis before 9 years of age, a congruous joint, and minimal head and neck involvement.

Stulberg and associates[136] in a classic paper described five possible head shapes at the end of the healing phase and correlated these with long-term outcome. In groups I and II, the femoral head was spherical, and arthritis did not develop over a long-term follow-up (Figs. 18, *J*, and 20, *E* and *F*). In group III, the femoral head was not spherical nor was it truly flat, and the acetabulum was congruous with the head (Fig. 21, *H* and *I*). In group IV, there was true flattening of the head and acetabulum (Fig. 22, *J*). In groups III and IV, termed congruous incongruity, mild to moderate degenerative changes developed in late adulthood. In group V, there was loss of shape of the femoral head without any adaptation of the acetabulum, and those with incongruous incongruity had degenerative disease in early adulthood.

In 1984, McAndrew and Weinstein[143] reevaluated 35 patients with 37 affected hips that had been studied previously by Gower and Johnston. These patients were found out of a group of 112 patients treated between 1920 and 1940 at the University of Iowa.[118] The original treatment had been with spica casts changed every 2 months for between 1 and 23 months. The average follow-up was 47.7 years. In this follow-up, almost half of the hips had been treated with arthroplasty for degenerative disease. Eleven arthroplasties had been done in the fifth or sixth decade of life, and four (three patients) were done in the third or fourth decade. Only 40% of hips had good function (with more than 80 points on the Iowa hip scale). Factors associated with poor outcome included presence of two or more of Catterall's risk factors, age of onset of over 8 years, and coxa magna. The Catterall classification did not correlate with outcome. Spherical heads did well without degenerative changes. McAndrew and Weinstein[143] concluded that half the patients with Legg-Calvé-Perthes disease will require hip replacement if followed into their fifth decade of life and that the only guarantee of a good result is a spherical femoral head. The major limitations of the study are that all patients received significant early treatment, which may have altered the outcome in either direction, and that a cohort of 35 cases out of an original 112 may not represent a true spectrum of the disease.

Several studies address the natural history at the ends of the spectrum of age at onset. Snyder[144] studied 31 hips in patients with onset younger than 5 years of age and found that ten of 31 had poor results. Some hips tended to improve in sphericity over the period from early healing to final follow-up. Snyder[144] mentions an unpublished work by Urban with 43% poor results in patients younger than 5 years old at onset. Ippolito and associates[145] studied patients with onset of disease during adolescence. The age at diagnosis was between 13 and 15 years with a follow-up that averaged 27.6 years. All patients developed pain and decreased range of motion between the end of treatment and 39 years of age, and two had radical surgical procedures. Ten hips were radiographed in follow-up, and all had degenerative changes.

In some patients, failure to heal the central portion of the femoral head results in persistent symptoms due to osteochondritis dissecans.

Osterman and Lindholm[146] estimated that 6% of Legg-Calvé-Perthes patients develop this complication. Bowen and associates[147] found osteochondritis lesions in 14 of 465 patients and estimated the incidence at 3%.

Another sequela of the disorder is leg length discrepancy. Shapiro[148] found an average discrepancy of 2.14 cm. The contribution of treatment to the length discrepancy is uncertain; in this study, the tibial discrepancy correlated with the duration of treatment in a brace.

Another approach toward understanding the natural history has been to determine the number of patients with osteoarthritis of the hip who had prior Legg-Calvé-Perthes disease. Solomon[149] studied patterns of osteoarthritis of the hip and surmised that one of three might be old Legg-Calvé-Perthes disease. Harris[150] found that more than 90% of patients with osteoarthritis of the hip had abnormalities suggestive of old slipped epiphysis, acetabular dysplasia, Legg-Calvé-Perthes disease, or other diseases such as epiphyseal dysplasia. Cooperman and associates[151] reported that most hip joint degenerative arthritis resulted from three childhood diseases: juvenile rheumatoid arthritis, Legg-Calvé-Perthes disease, and postreduction osteonecrosis in congenital hip dislocation.

Two studies have focused on patients who did poorly. Clarke and Harrison[152] reported 31 patients with an average age of 17 years who had painful hips after Legg-Calvé-Perthes disease. Half the patients had premature closure of the capital physis, and 54% had a mushroom head. Poussa and associates[129] studied 25 hips with a poor outcome out of 126 treated with varus osteotomy and found five early radiologic features associated with a poor prognosis. These included calcification lateral to the femoral head, widening of the femoral head before fragmentation, the saturn phenomenon (a dense central area of the capital epiphysis surrounded by lucency), early widening of the femoral neck, and early sclerotic changes in the metaphysis.

Finally, Herring and associates[153] note that the shape of the femoral head frequently continues to evolve in the period from early reossification to skeletal maturity (Figs. 21 and 24). Forty-nine of 136 hips studied became progressively more spherical, while in 15 there was progressive flattening over a 4-year period following reossification. These data emphasize the need to study patients until skeletal maturity before assessing the result of the disease or the effect of treatment

IMAGING

PLAIN RADIOGRAPHY

The discovery of Legg-Calvé-Perthes disease was catalyzed by the development of the X-ray machine in 1895. Radiographs of affected hips taken in 1905 have been discovered, and all the describers of the disorder were able to isolate it from tuberculosis primarily by its characteristic radiographic features. Waldenström first defined the stages of progression of the disease in 1920, and his classification is still valid and widely used.

Findings

Stages of Disease Progression Waldenström[95] described four stages in the evolution of radiographic changes in the femoral head. He stated that the initial stage of the evolutionary period lasts 6 to 12 months, during which the femoral head density gradually increases. Density changes in the metaphysis appear and later resolve. He believed that the fragmentation stage of the evolutionary period lasts for 2 to 3 years. The evolutionary period is followed by the healing period, which lasts for between 1 and 2 years as the head gradually reossifies. The third period, the growing period, lasts until growth is complete. The fourth period was called the definite stage. In common usage, four radiographic stages are ascribed to Waldenström; these are the initial, fragmentation, reossification, and healed stages (Figs. 21 and 22).[154] A five-stage classification probably covers the disorder best, with the stages being initial, increased density, fragmentation, reossification, and healed.

Initially Waldenström[155] and later Caffey[156] stated that the first sign of Legg-Calvé-Perthes disease was slight lateralization of the femoral head in the acetabulum. Synovitis and hypertrophy of articular cartilage have been suggested as the cause of this apparent widening of the medial joint space. Cartilage hypertrophy has been confirmed in several pathologic specimens.[57] More recently, Kamegaya[157] used enhanced computed tomography (CT) to show that early lateralization was due to swelling of the ligamentum teres.

Ferguson[158] noted that cessation of growth of the capital epiphysis was the first radiographic change. These two findings, lateralization of the head and a slightly smaller ossific nucleus, are generally considered to be the earliest findings on plain radiographs. The diagnosis may be made earlier using other techniques such as ultrasound, MRI, and scintigraphy. Swelling of the hip capsule had been stated to be a reliable early radiographic finding, but Brown[159] disputed this concept. He found that the appearance of capsular swelling was really due to a positioning artifact in which the film is taken with the hip abducted and laterally rotated.

As the first stage of the disease evolves, several subsequent changes occur. A linear fracture in the subchondral region of the femoral head is present very early in about a third of cases, and is termed Waldenström's sign. This is often best seen in the frog lateral projection.[155,156] Rarely, the fracture will fill with gas on the frog lateral radiograph; this reaction is presumed to be caused by a vacuum phenomenon that produces intra-articular gas on forced frog lateral views. An additional sign of early disease is a slight increase in density of the ossific nucleus seen only on the lateral projection.[156]

The second radiographic stage is that of increased density. During this stage, the entire ossific nucleus generally becomes radiodense, regardless of the extent of subsequent head collapse (Fig. 22).[95,156] The increase in density results from the accretion of new bone on the dead bone trabeculae of the ossific nucleus.[56,158] Studies by Herring and associates[153] have shown this stage to last a mean of 6 months, with a maximum duration of 14 months. Hips with more severe disease had a longer duration of each radiographic stage. During the increased density stage, ill-defined lucencies as well as sharply defined cysts appear in the metaphysis. This stage concludes when lucencies appear within the ossific nucleus.

The third radiographic stage is the fragmentation stage (Fig. 21, D and E).[96] During this stage, a portion of the femoral ossific nucleus becomes lucent while areas of sclerosis remain. The lucent areas evolve rapidly over several months, with the stage lasting from 2 to 35 months with a mean of 8 months.[153] During the fragmentation stage, the extent of major involvement of the femoral head becomes evident. There usually is

a central dense fragment that becomes demarcated from the medial and lateral portions of the head.[156] In more severe cases, there is no demarcation between the central and lateral segments, and there may or may not be a demarcation between the central and medial segments. The fragmentation stage concludes with new bone appearing in the subchondral areas of the femoral head. In mild cases, fragmentation may be seen only on the frog lateral radiograph, while there is a slightly mottled density on the anteroposterior (AP) radiograph. This observation suggests that the necrosis is isolated to the anterior portion of the epiphysis. In the mildest cases there is no true fragmentation stage at all, and the head begins to heal with gradual resolution of the dense areas.

The healing stage of the disorder begins with the appearance of subchondral new bone in the femoral head (Figs. 22, J, and 24, *top right*). This ossification often begins in the central portion of the head and spreads medially and laterally. The last portion to reossify is usually either the anterior portion (seen on the frog lateral film) or the central portion of the head. Gradually, the lucent areas of the head fill in with woven bone. The new bone gradually remodels to trabecular bone. The healing stage, which ends when the entire head is reossified, lasts from 2 to 122 months with a mean duration of 51 months. This stage is especially prolonged in more severely involved hips. It was previously thought that the femoral head shape changed little during this phase, but recent studies showed that most hips have gradual improvement of roundness over the several year duration of the healing stage.[153] A small minority of hips will have gradual flattening of the femoral head. This flattening tends to occur in children who are younger than 5 years of age at onset and have total head involvement.

The final phase of the disease is the residual stage.[95] In this stage there is no further evolution of femoral head density, but the contour of the femoral head may continue to evolve. Only at the end of growth is the contour of the head permanent.[153] The healed femoral head may vary from perfectly normal to extremely flattened and irregular. If there has been a growth disturbance of the capital physis, there may be progressive relative overgrowth of the greater trochanter during this period.

Bilateral Changes Bilateral density changes within the femoral head may or may not be Legg-Calvé-Perthes disease. Nevelös[160] noted four different patterns of bilateral disease. In type 1, the radiographic changes are similar in both hips and progress identically. These patients probably have a form of multiple epiphyseal dysplasia, and other epiphyses should be examined to confirm the diagnosis (Fig. 16). In type 2, the changes occur simultaneously on both sides but only one side fragments. In type 3, there are typical early findings in one hip in the presence of healed changes in the other hip. In type 4, the two hips are involved sequentially, with the last hip having the more severe course. The last two types are typical for Legg-Calvé-Perthes.

Other Features

Metaphyseal Changes There is considerable controversy about the nature and significance of radiographic changes in the metaphyseal area adjacent to the involved capital epiphysis. Gill[161] noted in 1940 that metaphyseal changes were evident very early in the disease process. He termed them "holes of decalcification," and believed that the femoral head changes resulted from necrosis in the metaphysis. Ponseti[162] found tongues of fibrillated cartilage extending deep into the femoral neck that caused the radiographic appearance of cystic changes in the neck. Katz and Siffert[163] believed that the cysts were due to resorption associated with revascularization as healing was occurring. They reported that poor results occurred twice as often in hips with cysts as in those without cystic change.

Hoffinger and associates[164,165] questioned the concept that the cysts are located purely within the metaphysis, and their work supports the concept of Ponseti that the lucencies represent extensions of the physeal cartilage into the metaphysis. In their study, 24 MRI scans were reviewed blindly and compared to the plain radiographs of the hip. Eleven of 23 hips with radiographic "cysts" had no metaphyseal changes on MRI, 12 had changes in the anterior metaphysis connecting to the physis, and one had a discrete metaphyseal cyst. They concluded that most metaphyseal cysts are really located within the epiphysis or physis and appear to be in the metaphysis as a projection artifact (Fig. 25).[164,165] There are a few cysts that truly are within the metaphysis.[166] Katz and

Siffert[163] felt that the metaphyseal changes were of prognostic significance. They noted that 49% of patients with poor results had metaphyseal cysts whereas only 26% of those with good results had such findings.

Physeal Changes Abnormal growth of the proximal femoral physis often occurs in hips with Legg-Calvé-Perthes disease. True epiphyseal bridging usually is not seen, and there are no good early signs of likely growth disturbance. Apley and Wientroub[167] described the "sagging rope" sign, a radiodense line overlying the proximal femoral metaphysis, caused by damage to the growth plate with marked metaphyseal reaction (Fig. 26). Keret and associates[168] reported an incidence of premature physeal closure of 25% in their patients, a much higher figure than found in other reports. Physeal closure was inferred when there was overgrowth of the greater trochanter, change in physeal shape, lateral protrusion of the capital nucleus, and medial bowing of the femoral neck. Barnes[169] reviewed 22 patients with evidence of early epiphyseal closure and found that the concomitant trochanteric overgrowth was not associated with a Trendelenburg gait. Bowen and associates[170] noted several types of deformity associated with physeal arrest. Central arrests produced a short femoral neck, round head, and overgrowth of the greater trochanter. Lateral closure resulted in a laterally tilted femoral head with a longer medial neck and an overgrown trochanter. Physeal arrest was noted to be a contraindication to femoral osteotomy. Sponseller and associates[171] found only three of 52 hips studied had evidence of definite premature closure of the physis. Many hips had deformity due to altered growth velocity, but true physeal bar formation was not seen. Langenskiöld[172] noted that there was a specific metaphyseal bulge, or step-shaped irregularity, seen on the lateral radiograph, that was similar to changes seen in Blount's disease. These were sometimes associated with early physeal closure. He recommended trochanteric arrest when early physeal closure was seen.

Acetabular Changes Changes in shape of the femoral head are almost always accompanied by parallel changes in the acetabulum. As the head extrudes from the acetabulum, the medial wall may remodel to form what appears to be a second

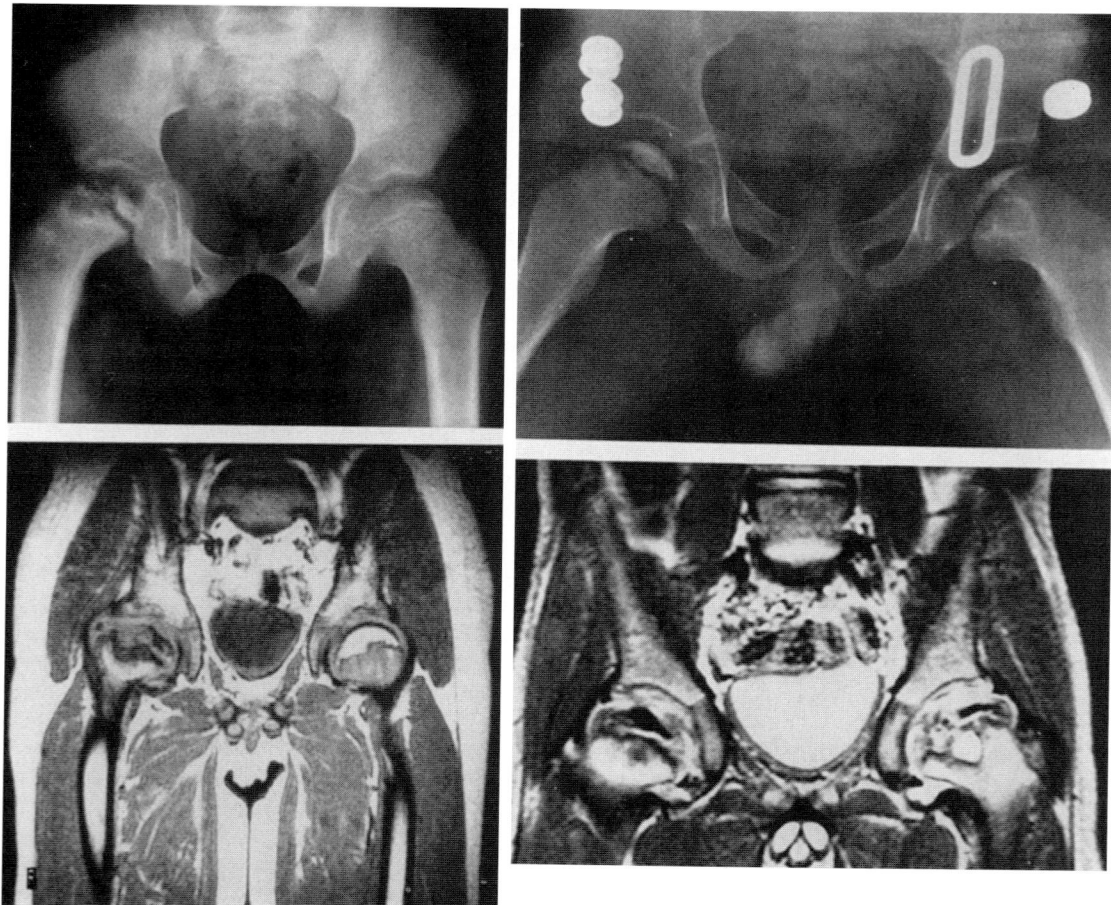

FIGURE 25
Left, An MRI (bottom) and corresponding radiograph (top) of a patient with diffuse metaphyseal reaction. The MRI demonstrates that the reaction is actually in the physis and appears metaphyseal as a radiographic artifact. **Right,** An MRI (bottom) with corresponding radiograph (top) showing a true metaphyseal cyst, which is fluid filled. (Reproduced with permission from Hoffinger SA, Henderson RC, Renner JB, et al: Magnetic resonance evaluation of metaphyseal changes in Legg-Calvé-Perthes disease. *J Pediatr Orthop* 1993;13:602-606.)

compartment for the femoral head. This was termed "bicompartmentalization" by Yngve and Roberts,[173] and was considered to be a sign of poor prognosis (Fig. 22). This sign was seen in 19 of 61 cases and was present as early as 3 months after onset. Joseph[174] also noted bicompartmental changes and believed they usually were associated with premature closure of the triradiate cartilage. He also noted that osteoporosis of the acetabular roof, which was present in the earliest stages of the disease, was maximum during the middle stages, with return to normal at skeletal maturity. Kamegaya and associates[175] noted that the position of the femoral head rather than sphericity was the most important factor in acetabular growth and remodeling. I have found that acetabular bicompartmentalization often will resolve during the healing phase of the disease (Fig. 21).

Minimal Changes
Meyer[176] reported a series of cases in which mild changes in the femoral head were found on incidental radiographs. These changes produced no

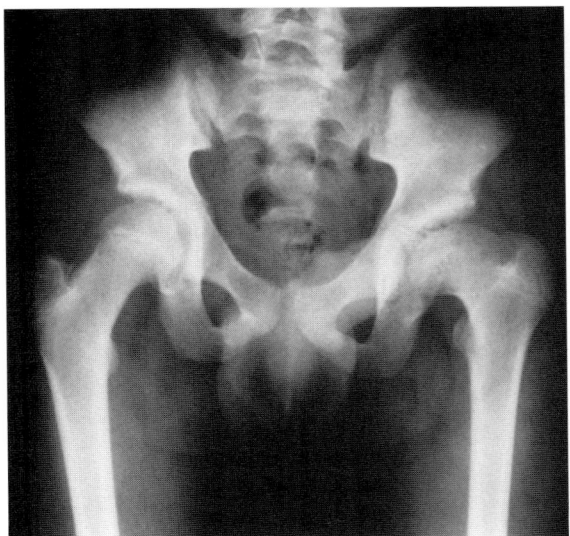 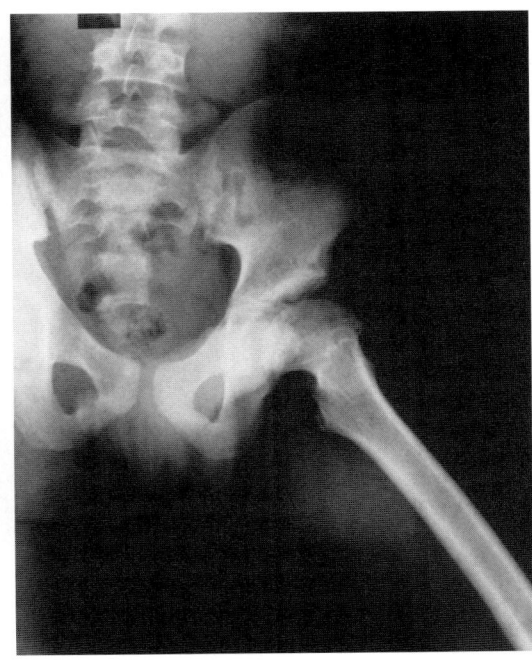

FIGURE 26
"Sagging rope" sign. **Left,** An anteroposterior (AP) radiograph showing a curvilinear density on the upper intertrochanteric area, the sagging rope. **Right,** A frog lateral radiograph showing the mushroom deformation of the femoral head that overlaps the metaphysis to produce the apparent sagging rope on the AP view.

permanent changes in head shape, and he believed this was a primary dysplasia of the hip rather than an osteonecrosis. This condition was termed Meyer's dysplasia, but probably represents asymptomatic osteonecrosis in a very young patient population.

Herring and associates[177] reported a series of 24 cases with radiographic changes that were limited to a small area of the femoral head. Ten had changes in the anterior segment, seven in the posteromedial portion, three in the lateral segment, and four in the central portion of the femoral head (Fig. 20). These changes evolved over time, and all femoral heads lost some height compared with the contralateral hip. The authors believed that these represented a very minor form of Legg-Calvé-Perthes, with the specific anatomic locations possibly related to segmental patterns of blood supply to the femoral head. Arie and associates[41] noted minor changes in the contralateral hip in patients with unilateral Legg-Calvé-Perthes disease. These hips were less round than normal with anterior flattening.

ARTHROGRAPHY

Arthrography allows visualization of the shape of the femoral head and the relationship of the head to the acetabulum. The necessity for arthrography remains controversial, and similar information may be obtained from the MRI scan (Figs. 22 and 27). Axer and Schiller[178] noted an increase in the medial joint space on arthrography in five of eight hips. This space averaged 3 mm and accompanied a lateral shift of the femoral head. Gershuni and associates[179] found thickening of the articular cartilage but no true medial joint space. They believed that lateralization of the femoral head occurred because of thickening of articular cartilage and change of femoral head shape. Contact between the head and acetabulum was always maintained, and there was no true subluxation in the early stage of the disease. Crawford and Carothers[180] reported the use of arthrography in 146 cases, noting that there were no complications and three unsuccessful attempts. They noted that the study provided accurate information about containment of the femoral head within the acetabulum. Gallagher and associates,[181] however, found that plain radiography provided sufficient information to evaluate extrusion of the femoral head, especially if the acetabulum-head quotient was used. They concluded that routine arthrography was not necessary to manage the disorder. Probably, the commonest use of arthrography is to diagnose the presence of hinge abduction (Fig. 27).

ULTRASONOGRAPHY

Ultrasonography is useful in the early stages of Legg-Calvé-Perthes disease to document joint effusion, and later to evaluate femoral head shape. Suzuki and associates[182] found that the outline of the cartilaginous femoral head was well seen and was similar to that found with arthrography. They were able to use ultrasound to follow femoral head deformation without the use of radiographs. Naumann[183] proposed a four-stage classification using ultrasound, and suggested that patients could be reliably followed without the use of radiographs.

TECHNETIUM SCANNING

Scintigraphy is useful for making the diagnosis of Legg-Calvé-Perthes disease before radiographic changes are evident. Several authors have also proposed scintigraphic classifications that may have prognostic value (Fig. 28). Wingstrand and associates[59] studied 25 cases of synovitis of the hip with negative radiographs and found four

that had markedly decreased uptake of isotope by the epiphysis. When studied 6 weeks later, only one hip had a persistent defect of uptake of tracer, and that hip developed Legg-Calvé-Perthes disease. Fasting and associates[184] graded the severity of involvement by scintigraphy into four grades ranging from grade I, (one fourth of the epiphysis involved) to grade IV (total epiphyseal involvement). Oshima and associates[185] compared three-phase scintigraphy to single photon emission computed tomography (SPECT) and to MRI. Increased activity was present in the epiphysis or physis in 39% of cases, with 94% having increased uptake on the blood-pool images. A lateral stripe of revascularization was seen with pinhole images in 57% of patients. Cross-sectional views provided by SPECT gave a three-dimensional picture of femoral head necrosis. Conway[186] noted that scintigraphy could distinguish the physiology of the revascularization process. He found that recanalization occurred rapidly in the early stages of the disorder and could be distinguished from neovascularization, which is a prolonged process. He proposed two tracks: the A track, in which recanalization is present, with a short duration of healing and good prognosis, and the B track, with slow neovascularization and a poor prognosis. He also described a third process in which complications of the healing process, such as collapse and extrusion, occur, and during which the hip may revert from one track to the other.

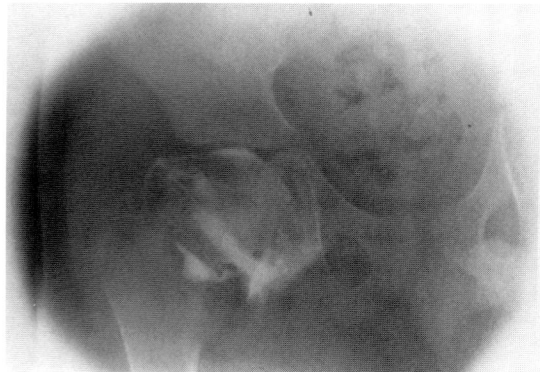 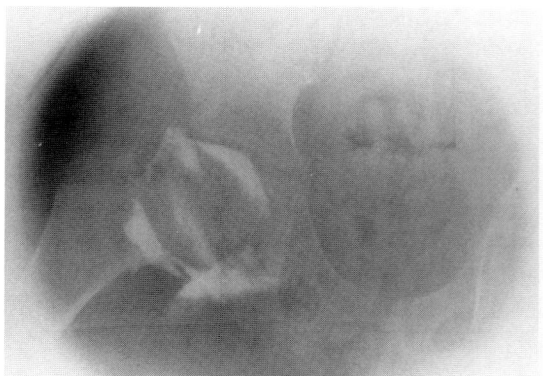

FIGURE 27

An example of "hinge abduction." **Left,** An arthrogram showing flattening of the femoral head and acetabulum with the hip in a neutral position. **Right,** The same hip in abduction. The femoral head hinges out of the acetabulum leaving a triangular dye filled cavity within the joint. In the fragmentation stage, this deformity may resolve with containment treatment. In the healed stage it is unlikely to improve.

MAGNETIC RESONANCE IMAGING

MRI scanning is probably the best tool for early diagnosis and for determining the shape of the femoral head and acetabulum (Fig. 25). Pinto and associates[187] reported two cases in which radiographs and bone scans were negative, and the MRI provided the early diagnosis. Theissen and associates[188] found that the accuracy of diagnosis was 88% to 93% for radiography, 88% to 91% for scintigraphy, and 97% to 99% for MRI. On the other hand, Elsig and associates[189] reported a case in which the MRI was normal while the technetium scan showed early osteonecrosis. As early as 1984, Scoles and associates[190] were able to produce arthrogram-like images with MRI. Grimm and associates[191] found that MRI could show the congruity of articular surfaces, femoral head containment, joint effusion, and hypertrophy of the synovium. They noted that lateralization of the femoral head was due to medial hypertrophy of the head cartilage. They also reported that the state of revascularization could be determined. Ranner and associates[192] reported that MRI gave as early a diagnosis as bone scanning, but believed that in follow-up the scan was better in showing the start of revascularization. Henderson and asociates[193] reported that MRI better delineated the extent and location of areas of involvement in the early stages of the disease. Egund and Wingstrand[194] compared MRI with arthrography and found that the MRI gave more information about the medial and lateral aspects of the cartilaginous capital epiphysis. Bos and associates[195] performed sequential MRI studies and found a correlation with the Catterall classification. In Catterall group II hips, there was considerable viable bone medially, laterally, and posteriorly. In group III there was more extensive necrosis, and group IV had involvement of the growth plate with repair going into the metaphysis. Kumasaka and associates[196] devised an epiphyseal index for MRI studies, and defined the normal index to be 0.39 to 0.60. The average for affected hips was 0.31 in the fragmentation stage and 0.31 in the residual stage.

COMPUTERIZED TOMOGRAPHY

CT scanning is not routinely used in Legg-Calvé-Perthes disease. Accurate three-dimensional information about the contour of the femoral head and acetabulum can be obtained.[197-199] Moreno and associates[199] classified the findings into three groups: group A with limited peripheral involvement, group B with extensive central necrosis but no posterior involvement, and group C with whole head involvement. Although it may be useful for certain purposes, clinical decisions are usually not based on early CT scan information.

CT often is helpful in evaluating the patient with pain, locking, and other mechanical symptoms that begin years after the initial episode of Legg-Calvé-Perthes. Scans of the femoral head may differentiate between a loose fragment and an area of incomplete reossification within the femoral head.

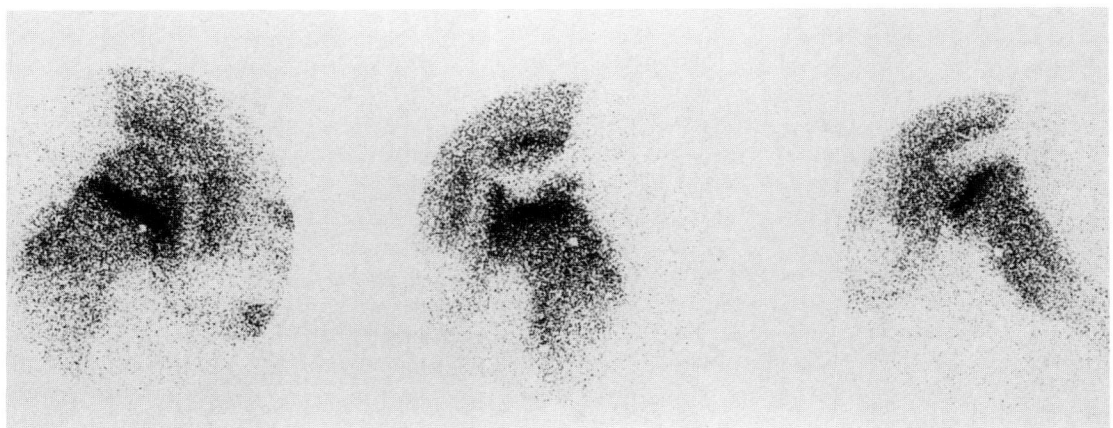

FIGURE 28
A technetium scan of a patient with Legg-Calvé-Perthes of the left hip. **Left,** There is normal uptake in the right hip. **Center** and **Right,** The two views of the left hip show absence of uptake in the central portion of the femoral head.

TREATMENT

SYMPTOMATIC TREATMENT

Bed rest and traction are the mainstays of symptomatic treatment, and nonsteroidal anti-inflammatory medications are a useful adjunct. The use of crutches for reduced weightbearing also may be helpful. No formal studies of bed rest are available, but parents of affected children often discover its beneficial effects on their own. Especially in the early phases of the disease, a day of bed rest will reduce pain and increase the range of motion of the hip; this improvement is presumed to result from a reduction of synovitis. This effect is maximal about the time of the appearance of the subchondral fracture. Later in the disease, during the fragmentation and reossification phases, loss of range of motion may be a result of femoral head deformity, and bed rest will not restore motion.

Traction is used in several ways. Simple longitudinal traction applied to the affected leg with 4

or 5 lbs of weight attached to the child's bed at home may be helpful. The traction may be used at night only, either every night or only when pain and spasm are present, or it may be used all day for several days or weeks until the range of motion improves. Traction in the hospital may also be used, and various methods have been employed. Some use simple longitudinal traction with the leg on the bed, while others use balanced suspension and traction, or "slings and springs," and either method may be used to gradually abduct the affected extremity (Fig. 29).

Several studies support the use of traction and help specify the optimal hip position during traction. Kallio and Ryöppy[91] measured intra-articular pressure in 94 hips of children with various forms of synovitis and found mild elevation of pressure in patients with Legg-Calvé-Perthes disease. The pressure within the hip was lowest in a position of 30° to 45° of flexion and slight external rotation. When traction was applied with the hip in full extension, there was a marked increase in

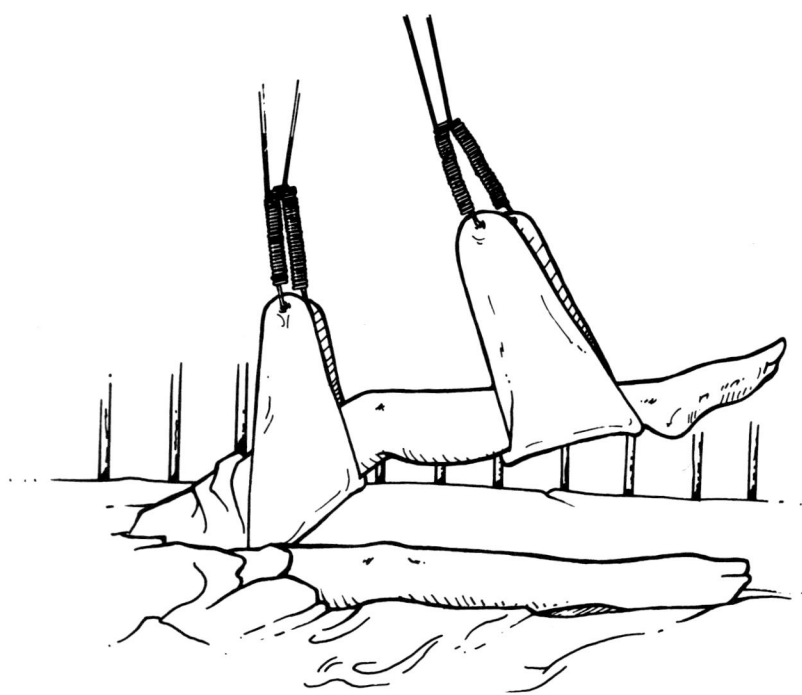

FIGURE 29
"Slings and springs," which prove to be useful and simple in regaining range of motion of an irritable hip.

intra-articular pressure, suggesting that this position should not be used in children with synovitis of the hip of any origin. Serlo and associates[200] also studied intra-articular pressure in Legg-Calvé-Perthes disease and found that 7 to 14 days of Russel's traction decreased the intra-articular pressure significantly and increased hip range of motion a mean of 34°. In addition, they showed a significant reduction of venous congestion using osteovenography. Naito and associates[201] studied blood flow in canine femoral heads while applying an experimental joint tamponade. They found that traction at one half body weight did not affect blood flow to the femoral head, but a traction force equal to body weight markedly compromised blood flow to the femoral head.

Crutches and partial or nonweightbearing are frequently used to reduce pain and improve range of motion, but there are no specific studies of this modality. In fact the difficulty of keeping a child from weightbearing when using crutches resulted in the introduction of the Snyder sling.[18] Currently, long-term use of crutches is not recommended.

CONTAINMENT TREATMENT

Rationale and Experimental Basis

Salter,[202] in an abstract published in 1966, briefly described a series of experiments conducted using pigs in which avascular necrosis of the femoral head was produced by ligation of the arterial supply, by injection of vessels, and by application of continuous pressure to the femoral head. He noted that the first radiologic sign of osteonecrosis was failure of the ossified part of the head to grow while there was continued growth of the cartilage model. The newly formed bone was deformed when the hip remained in a neutral or adducted position. When weightbearing was allowed with the hip in flexion and abduction, the acetabulum served as a mold, and the femoral head did not become deformed.

Two years later, Salter and Bell[203] described placing the pigs with osteonecrosis into three groups: one group was allowed normal weightbearing, a second was held in acute flexion of the hip to prevent weightbearing, and a third was placed into abduction with weightbearing allowed. Only the third group had round femoral heads, suggesting again that containment within the acetabulum prevented femoral head deformation. They termed this response biologic plastici-

ty. This containment concept has replaced the older concept of inexorable physical softening of the necrotic head.

Salter[22] later elaborated his concept of the pathogenesis of deformity. He noted that the disorder begins with femoral head ischemia, which is followed by revascularization. During revascularization, the femoral head is vulnerable to a pathologic subchondral fracture. This fracture fails to unite, with subsequent resorption of underlying bone and collapse of the head. Then the head flattens, and a portion of it extrudes anterolaterally out of the acetabulum. The edge of the acetabulum now exerts excessive pressure on the softened femoral head, which further flattens and deforms.

A number of methods to "contain" the femoral head within the acetabulum have evolved; these methods include bracing, Petrie cast wear, innominate osteotomy, femoral osteotomy, and acetabular shelf procedures. Rab and associates[133] performed a finite element analysis of femoral head stresses and found that if only the central portion of the femoral head was necrotic, the remaining lateral rim of bone would stress shield the central core and prevent collapse. When there was extensive necrosis, the shielding effect was lost and the head collapsed. They noted that while the femoral head represents 120% of a hemisphere, the acetabulum is only 75% of a hemisphere. Thus, only 63% of the head is in contact with the acetabulum at any time, and which portion of the head is covered is a function of the phase of gait as the joint moves. The study of varus osteotomy and innominate osteotomy configurations and the discovery that stresses were not reduced by these procedures led them to conclude that there was no mechanical basis for using containment osteotomies when there was extensive necrosis.

Rab[204] subsequently performed gait analyses on children with Legg-Calvé-Perthes disease to determine the dynamic effects of various containment devices. He found that Petrie casts produced increased anterior and lateral coverage while reducing posterior and medial coverage. The Atlanta brace produced hip flexion and external rotation, which added more posterior coverage than lateral coverage. He constructed a "containment index" and found that the Atlanta brace increased containment from a normal of 64% to 72%, whereas Petrie casts and the Toronto brace did not improve this index. Reimers[205] questioned whether any hips in children over 8 years of age are completely contained, a condition he defined as a migration percentage of 0%. He found that only 4% of hips with Legg-Calvé-Perthes and 10% of their contralateral, uninvolved hips were completely contained. In an earlier work, Reimers[206] found that only 22% of normal hips were completely contained in children between 8 and 12 years of age.

In spite of some skepticism, containment treatment has been clinically accepted and used for many years. The common methods of using this form of treatment will be described.

Nonsurgical Treatment A variety of orthoses have been designed for containment treatment of Legg-Calvé-Perthes disease. All of the braces abduct the involved hip, some control rotation, and most allow the hip to flex. Almost all authors stress the importance of regaining the range of motion of the irritable hip prior to beginning treatment, and the previously described methods of traction, bed rest, and reduced weightbearing are recommended for this purpose. The range of motion must be maintained throughout the treatment period, and in the more severe cases this may be difficult or impossible.

Petrie and Bitenc[207] in 1971 described the treatment of 60 patients with a program of traction or bed rest to achieve abduction of at least 45°. Adductor tenotomy was performed when necessary and the patients were placed in casts with bars between the legs abducting the hips to 45° and internally rotating them 5° to 10° (Fig. 6). The casts were changed each 3 to 4 months with mobilization of knees and ankles between casts. The treatment was continued until the femoral head was well into the healing phase, an average time in casts of 19 months. They reported 60% good, 31% fair, and 9% poor results using the Mose criteria. "Petrie casts" are still commonly used, especially when other methods fail. Richards and Coleman[208] reported using this method when there was painful limitation of motion that prevented proper positioning of the femoral head for brace wear. In these older children, it was necessary to apply the casts under general anesthesia, and adductor longus tenotomy was often necessary. Improved femoral head congruity was obtained after an average of 7 months of wearing the casts, which were changed each 3 months.

A series of braces named for the city of origin or for the originator have been used in various centers. The Birmingham brace and the Toronto brace were very complicated devices that are little used today. The Birmingham brace was a tribute to the obstinate pursuit of perfect immobilization (Fig. 30). The brace consisted of a leather corset, which reached from the nipple line to above the knee on the affected side, and had a kneeling bar and a chain to maintain the foot off the ground. A special crutch allowed the foot to clear while walking, and several padlocks that were opened only at the monthly clinic visits encouraged compliance.[20,209] The Toronto brace was unusually heavy and complex, because it was designed to maintain hip abduction in both a sitting and standing position. It was rumored that the universal joint at the base of the brace, which was an automotive universal joint, lasted longer in the family automobile than it did when worn by a child (Fig. 31).[210,211] Another heavy and complex device is the Newington orthosis, which consists of a metal A-frame with a central thigh support (Fig. 32).[212,213] Roberts[214] developed a brace made of leather that reproduced the position obtained in Petrie casts. Tachdjian and Jouett[215] designed a unilateral orthosis with an ischial seat that was fairly simple, but lacked purchase to maintain position in an irritable hip.

The most popular orthosis in current use is the Atlanta Scottish Rite orthosis (Fig. 33). The major advantage of this brace is that children rapidly regain the ability to walk and run, and resume many activities such as climbing trees and playing soccer and tennis. The brace consists of a metal waist band with hip hinges, thigh cuffs, and a telescoping rod between the thigh cuffs that allows abduction but limits adduction. The brace maintains the hips in abduction and the children usually walk with the hips flexed and externally rotated. As with other methods, obtaining and maintaining hip range of motion is an essential component of the treatment program. Purvis and associates[216] described the use of the Atlanta brace in 1980 and noted that 1 to 2 months of preliminary treatment to regain motion was necessary in more severely involved hips. They also noted that a return to traction was necessary if range of motion was lost during treatment. It was recommended that the orthosis be worn day and night. The patients were weaned from the brace when new bone formation was present on both

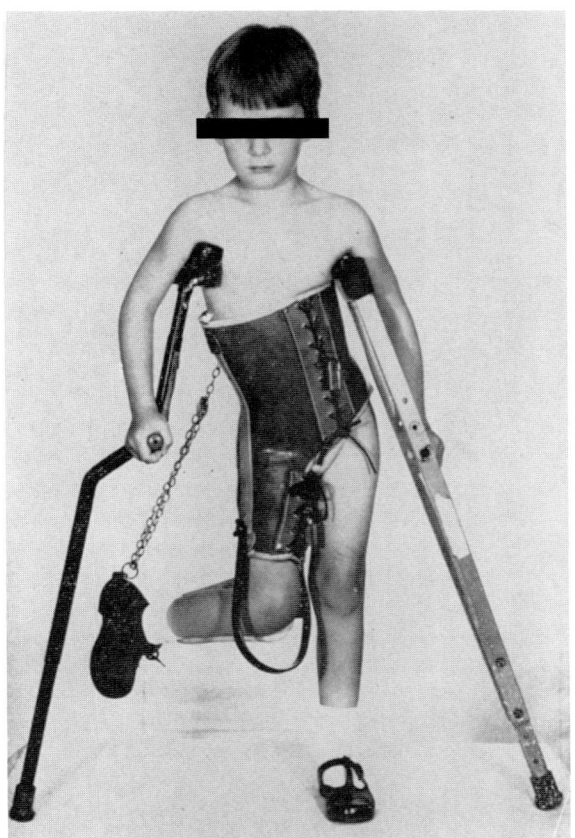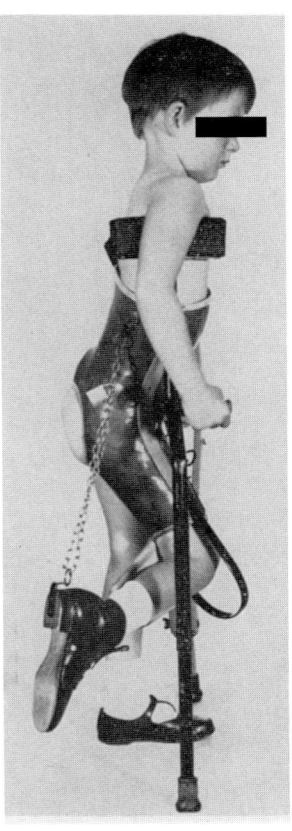

FIGURE 30
Left, The Birmingham brace, which has a kneeling bar and an altered crutch to allow clearance of the abducted, internally rotated limb. **Right,** The side view of the Birmingham brace demonstrates one of the three padlocks that kept the child in the orthosis until returning to the hospital for a bath. The nurse kept the key. (Reproduced with permission from Harrison MH, Turner MH, Smith DN: Perthes' disease: Treatment with the Birmingham splint. *J Bone Joint Surg* 1982;64B:3-11.)

AP and lateral radiographs, and the average duration of treatment was 18.9 months.

Current use of the Atlanta orthosis is often less rigorous than the program described by Purvis and associates. At the Texas Scottish Rite Hospital, an individualized program is used. In patients with milder disease, as judged by ease of maintaining range of motion as well as radiographic findings, the patient is allowed out of the brace at night. As the femoral head enters the fragmentation stage, if no collapse is noted and the lateral pillar is intact, part time bracing is begun and continued as long as a satisfactory range of motion is maintained. Bracing is discontinued when subchondral new bone formation is present on the AP radiograph. The usual duration of treatment is between 9 months and 1 year. In more

severely involved hips, full-time brace wear is necessary, and the range of motion must be maintained throughout the treatment period.

Surgical Treatment

Femoral Osteotomy Axer[217] in 1965 reported a series of cases in which he performed subtrochanteric femoral osteotomies for Legg-Calvé-Perthes disease, and he credited Somerville with having first done the procedure. Craig and associates[218] reported that most patients with Legg-Calvé-Perthes had excessive femoral anteversion and that they performed a femoral osteotomy to correct the excessive anteversion and an acetabuloplasty to improve acetabular coverage. They claimed that this treatment hastened the healing

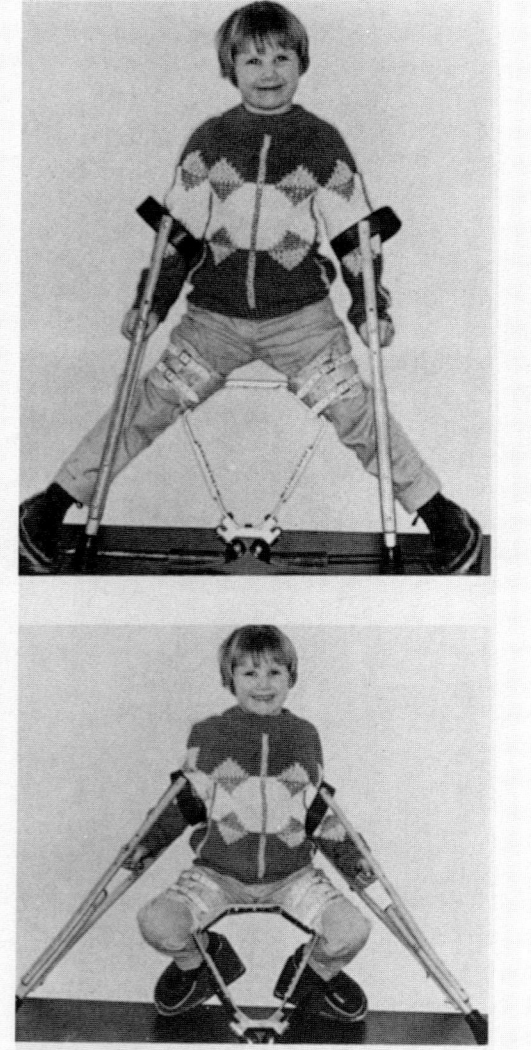

FIGURE 31
The Toronto Brace with its universal joints, which allow hip and knee flexion while maintaining hip abduction. (Reproduced with permission from Bobechko WP: The Toronto brace for Legg-Perthes disease. *Clin Orthop* 1974;102:115-117.)

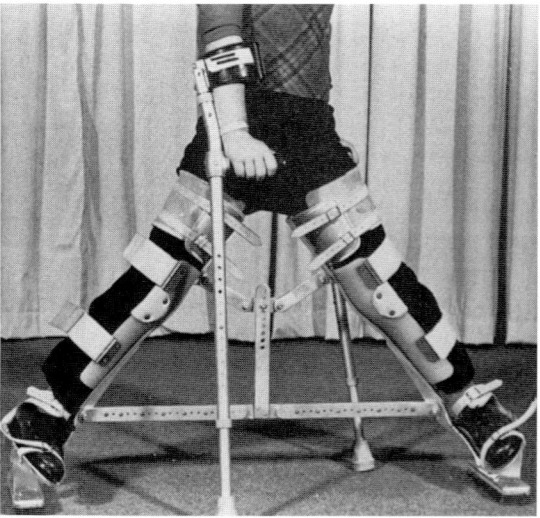

FIGURE 32
The Newington Brace which reproduces the hip position obtained with Petrie casts. (Reproduced with permission from Drennan JC: Orthotic management of Legg-Perthes disease, in Leach RE, Hoaglund FT, Riseborough EJ (eds): *Controversies in Orthopaedic Surgery.* Philadelphia, PA, WB Saunders, 1982, pp 315-325.)

of the osteonecrosis. Subsequently, many authors have reported good results from the use of varus, derotational femoral osteotomy in Legg-Calvé-Perthes disease (Fig. 34).

Several indications and prerequisites for femoral osteotomy in Legg-Calvé-Perthes disease are frequently mentioned. The indications most often cited are an age of onset over 6 years and a hip at risk for a poor result by some radiographic criteria. Surgery should be done before

the femoral head has begun to reossify. Lloyd-Roberts and associates[219] proposed that a femoral osteotomy was indicated for hips that had radiographic "at risk" signs without severe deformity of the femoral head. They suggested that the procedure be done within 8 months of the onset of symptoms. They found no improvement in outcome in children younger than 6 years of age at onset and recommended that those children be left untreated. McElwain and associates[220] required at least three "at risk" signs but operated on children as young as 3 years 6 months of age.

Most authors stress the importance of regaining hip motion prior to performing femoral osteotomy. Killian and Niemann[221] stressed the need for preoperative traction and used skeletal traction if skin traction failed to restore enough range of motion to "contain" the femoral head within the acetabulum. They were able to "contain" hips that were subluxated or that had "hinge abduction" by using preoperative skeletal traction to distract the joint and seat the head in the acetabulum. Others have used Petrie casts to regain range of motion. Lloyd-Roberts and associates[219] reported that the range of motion of the hip was usually improved under anesthesia and

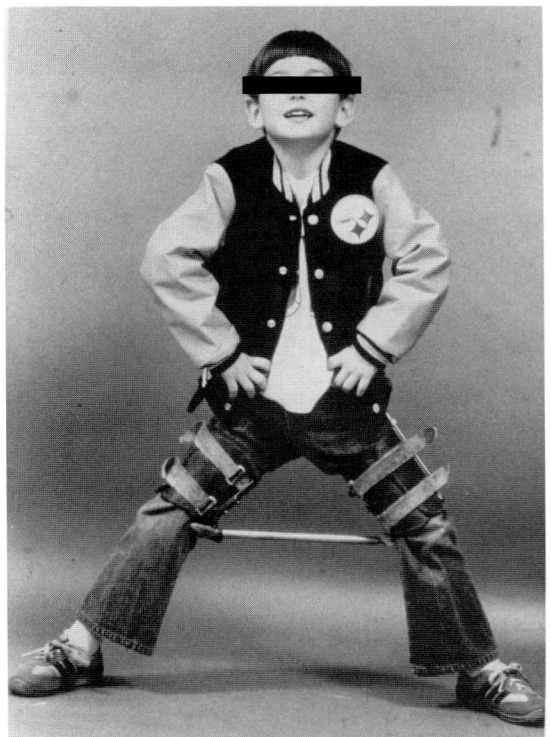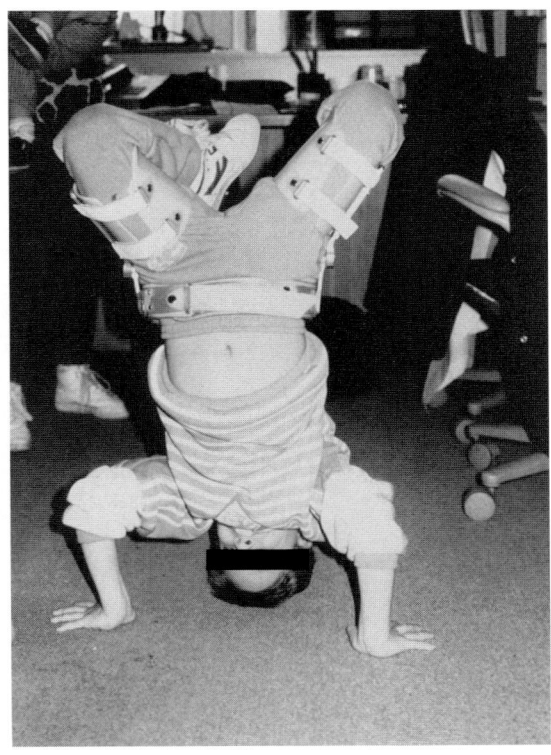

FIGURE 33
Left, An Atlanta Brace which consists of a pelvic band, hip hinges, thigh cuffs, and an extensile bar between the legs. **Right,** This view of the Atlanta Brace shows one of the activities possible in the orthosis. The advantage of this brace is that it allows considerable mobility.

that femoral osteotomy could be performed without prior traction.

Several authors have suggested that femoral osteotomy hastens the healing of the avascular process, but studies by other authors have refuted this concept. Clancy and Steel[222] and later Kendig and Evans[223] performed "biologic" osteotomies in which there was no displacement of the bone fragments and found no effect on the rate of healing of the avascular process. Marklund and Tillberg[224] found no difference in healing of the femoral heads when surgically treated hips were compared to nonsurgically-managed hips.

Barnes[169] reported 22 cases of Legg-Calvé-Perthes disease in which premature closure of the capital epiphysis had occurred, and implied that the femoral osteotomy may have caused the arrest. He concluded that this was more likely if the osteotomy was done after femoral head deformity was present. It also was more likely when the osteotomy was done in the earliest phases of the disease. Karpinski and associates[225] pointed out many disadvantages of femoral osteotomy, which included failure of the varus to remodel, shortening of the leg, increased abductor lurch, trochanteric overgrowth, and the need to remove the fixation device (Fig. 35). They found that the operation was detrimental to 30% of the Catterall group 1 hips and concluded that it was a mistake to surgically treat these milder cases. The degree of remodeling of the varus component depended on the ability of the capital physis to grow, a factor difficult to predict. An abductor limp was frequently present after femoral osteotomy, and they recommended trochanteric epiphysiodesis when trochanteric overgrowth was likely.

A number of aspects of the surgical technique of femoral osteotomy are controversial. Various authors recommend different degrees of varus and derotation to obtain containment of the femoral head. In Evans and associates'[121] series, the preoperative neck-shaft angles averaged 137°,

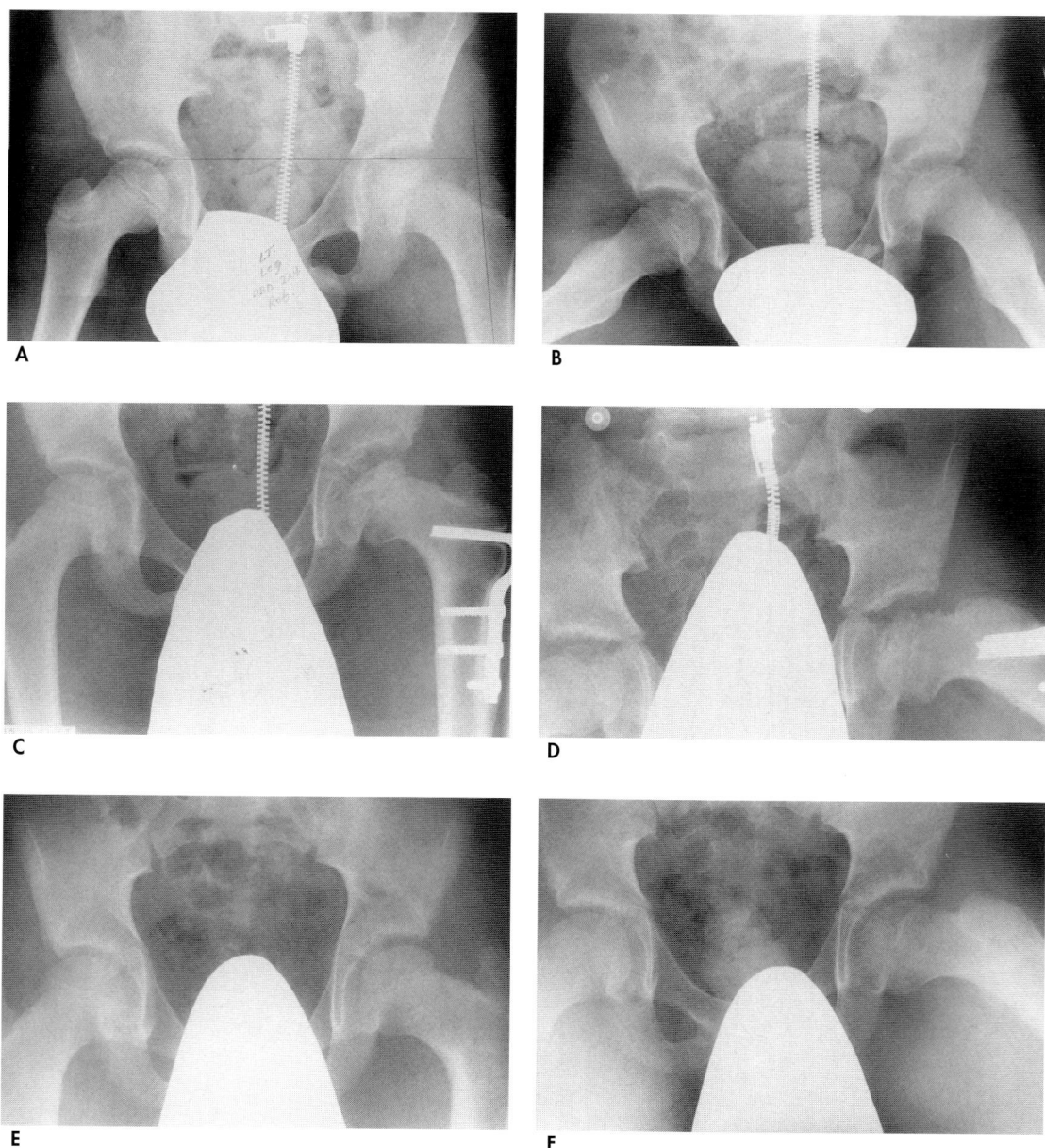

A

B

C

D

E

F

FIGURE 34

A 9-year 8-month old boy with recent onset of symptoms. He was treated with a femoral varus osteotomy. **A,** Initial antero-posterior (AP) radiograph showing a subchondral fracture extending over two thirds of the femoral head. **B,** Frog lateral radi-ograph at onset with an extensive subchondral fracture. **C,** AP radiograph 1 year after onset and 6 months after varus femoral osteotomy. The femoral head is well into reossification. **D,** A frog lateral radiograph 1 year after onset. The head is almost com-pletely reossified on this view. **E,** AP radiograph 4 years after onset. The femoral head is almost normal in contour and is com-pletely healed. **F,** Frog lateral radiograph showing a round femoral head, a Stulberg II result.

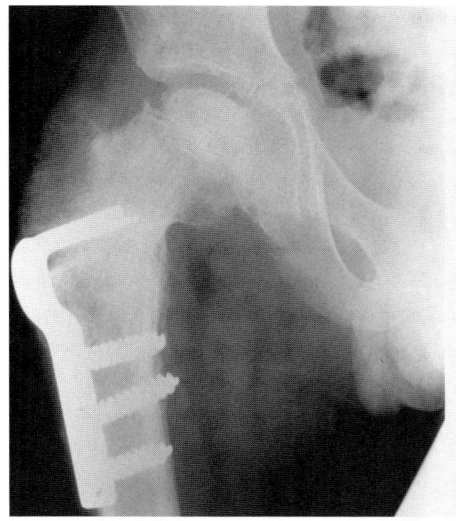
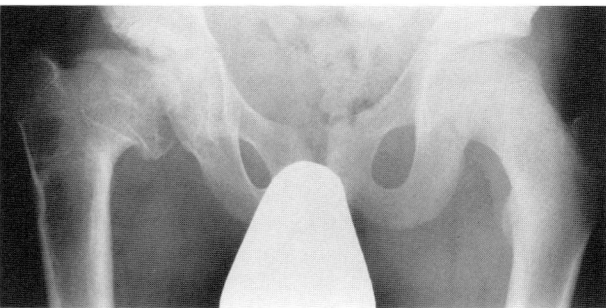
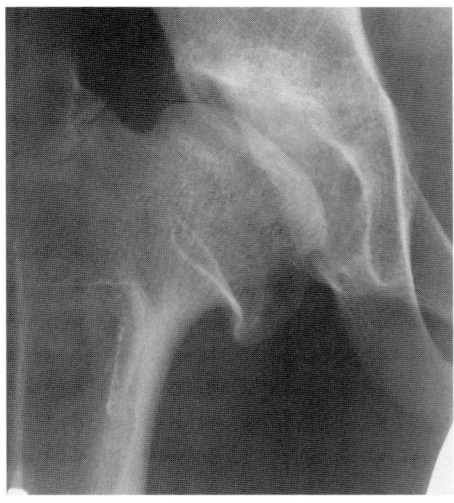
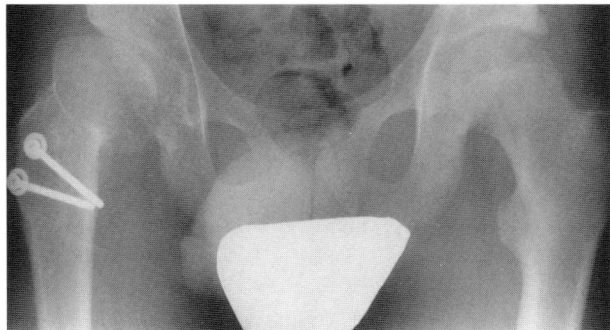

FIGURE 35

This 10-year-old boy was treated with a varus femoral osteotomy. **Top left,** Anteroposterior (AP) radiograph following femoral osteotomy. The greater trochanter is at the level of the femoral head. **Top right,** AP radiograph 2 years after onset. There appears to be closure of the central part of the capital femoral physis. **Bottom left,** AP radiograph 5 years after onset showing closure of the capital physis with overgrowth of the greater trochanter. The patient had a noticeable abductor limp. **Bottom right,** AP radiograph following transfer of the greater trochanter. The abductor limp was eliminated following this procedure.

the immediate postoperative angle was 116°, and the angle at final follow-up was 129°. They performed an unspecified amount of derotation in 14 of 19 hips. Heikkinen and Puranen[226] recommended producing a neck shaft angle of 100° to 110° and stated that this is not an excessive degree of varus because the neck tends to grow back into valgus. On the other hand, Weiner and associates[227] suggest that only enough varus to

barely position the femoral head beneath the lateral acetabular rim should be used, and never should the angle be less than 105°. Menelaus[228] recommended an extension, derotational osteotomy because it results in less residual femoral neck deformity. Laurent and Poussa[229] described adding 30° of varus regardless of the neck-shaft angle. Several authors have recommend performing an epiphysiodesis of the greater trochanter at the time of osteotomy or at plate removal to reduce trochanteric overgrowth.[121,228]

Complications of femoral osteotomy include shortening of the extremity, abductor limp, fracture after plate removal, excessive varus, and nonunion. Sponseller and associates[230] compared femoral and innominate osteotomy and found that femoral osteotomy caused greater shortening of the extremity. They also noted that an abductor limp was more common in the femoral osteotomy patients. Evans and associates[121] noted 20° to 30° loss of external rotation and 5° to 35° loss of abduction in patients treated with either femoral osteotomy or a brace. Their femoral osteotomy patients had an average of 2.1 surgical procedures, and 11% developed complications including delayed union, excessive varus, and wound infection. Excessive varus was corrected by a subsequent valgus osteotomy and several patients required epiphysiodesis for limb length discrepancy.

Leitch and associates[231] compared surgically and nonsurgically treated patients, and found that femoral osteotomy resulted in reduced articular trochanteric distance, which was associated with a Trendelenburg gait. Because this problem was common in older children, they recommended that the procedure not be performed in those over 8 years of age. Axer and associates[232] reported a series of femoral osteotomies in which seven of 70 hips had a second osteotomy because the first did not provide enough containment of the femoral head. Wenger[233] reported 18 cases of femoral osteotomy in which further collapse of the femoral head produced severe loss of range of motion. These hips required vigorous treatment with traction, muscle releases, and abduction cast or brace management. Finally, external rotation of the limb may be a persistent problem when a rotational osteotomy has been performed.

Innominate Osteotomy Based on the results of treatment of experimental osteonecrosis in pigs, Salter[234] first performed his innominate osteotomy for Legg-Calvé-Perthes disease in 1962. His prerequisites included minimal femoral head deformity as determined by arthrogram, no significant limitation of motion, and no irritability of the hip (Fig. 36).[22] His indications were an age of onset greater than 6 years, moderate or severe involvement, and loss of containment. He required that the hip abduct to 45° and the femoral head should

be contained in that position. He noted that preoperative treatment to regain range of motion was often required and included bed rest, traction, use of slings and springs, and at times surgical release of the adductor muscles with abduction casts for several weeks.[234]

Salter[234] recommended that the originally described surgical technique should be used, but emphasized that the capsule is not opened, and the iliopsoas must always be lengthened. He stated that when the adductor muscles are tight, they should be lengthened, and in most children a cast is not necessary if three heavy threaded pins are used to fix the osteotomy.

The Kalamchi modification of the Salter procedure is preferred by some surgeons.[235] This procedure repositions the distal pelvic fragment into a notch created posteriorly in the proximal side of the transected ilium. The purpose of the modification is to reposition the acetabulum without lengthening the pelvis to avoid increasing the pressure on the femoral head. Complications of innominate osteotomy include loss of fixation with displacement of the distal fragment, stiffness, lengthening of the extremity, and loss of hip flexion.[236]

Shelf Arthroplasty Shelf arthroplasty has been performed for the treatment of Legg-Calvé-Perthes disease since as early as 1940.[237] The indications for the procedure have included lateral subluxation of the femoral head, inadequate coverage of the femoral head, or hinge abduction of the hip, usually following other treatment modes. Kruse and associates[237] reported a series of cases in which the procedure was performed after an average of 2 years of nonsurgical treatment. Other authors have recommended the procedure as a primary containment method and have performed the procedure within 6 months of the onset of symptoms.[238]

Kruse performs the procedure described by Gill[239] in which a deep cut is made in the pelvis above the acetabulum to allow the acetabular roof to be "pried down." The shelf procedure described by Staheli and Chew[240] has also been used in Legg-Calvé-Perthes disease. Complications include an over-wide augmentation graft that causes loss of hip flexion and a thin graft that may fracture and fail to improve hip coverage. Dysesthesia of the lateral femoral cutaneous nerve also may complicate the procedure.

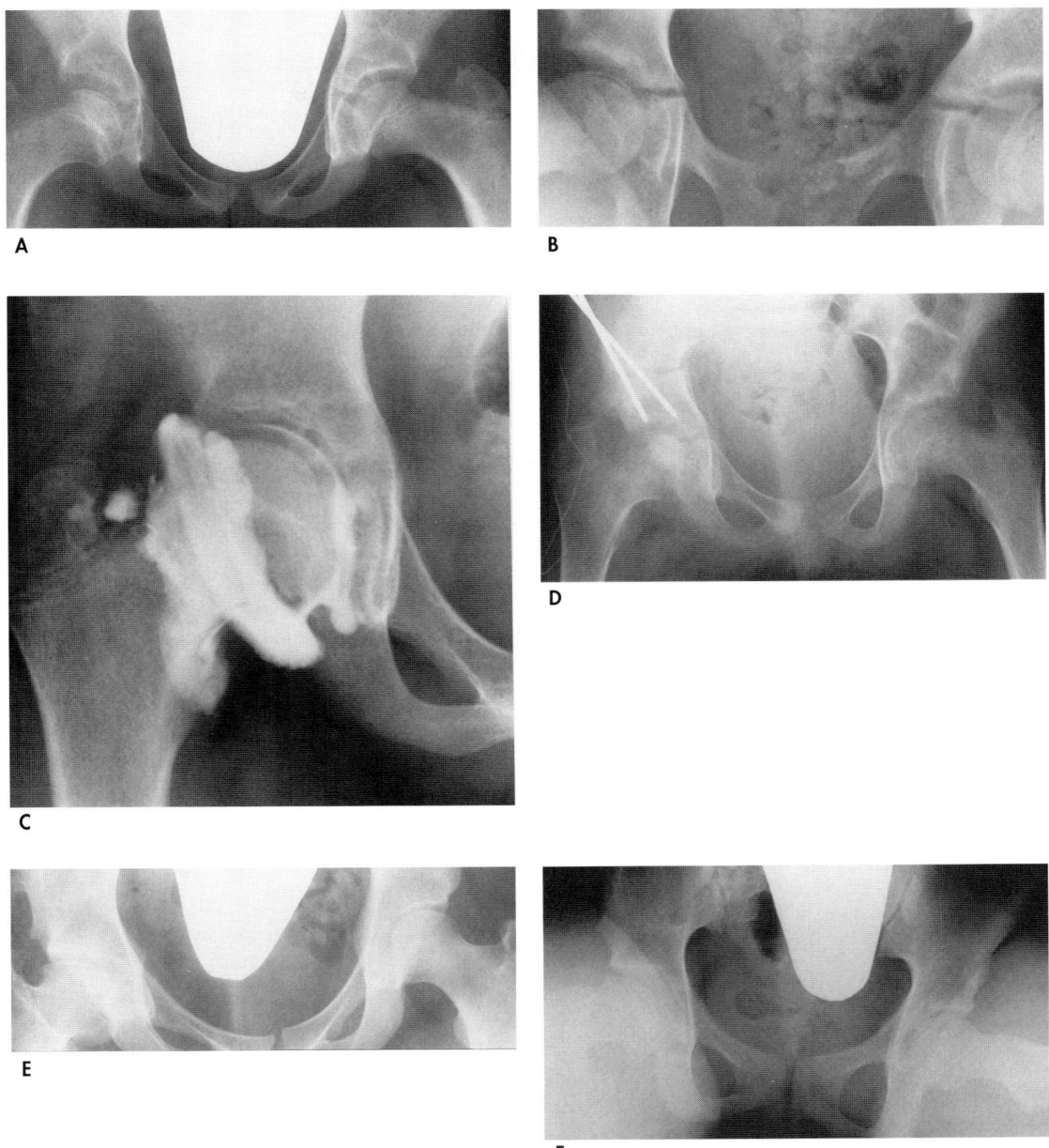

FIGURE 36

A 10-year-old girl with recent onset of Legg-Calvé-Perthes. A, Initial anteroposterior (AP) radiograph shows an extensive sub-chondral fracture line. B, Frog lateral radiograph shows a subchondral fracture involving the anterior two fifths of the head. C, An arthrogram at presentation shows no deformation of the femoral head. D, AP radiograph following innominate osteotomy. E, AP radiograph 8 years after osteotomy. The femoral head is fairly round and there is relative trochanteric overgrowth. F, A frog lateral radiograph 8 years after osteotomy shows a round femoral head, a Stulberg II result.

Combined Femoral and Innominate Osteotomy

Femoral osteotomy combined with innominate osteotomy has also been proposed to treat Legg-Calvé-Perthes.[241,242] The procedure is recommended for hips with a poor prognosis based on the presence of lateral subluxation, lateral calcification, and extensive metaphyseal changes. In these severely involved hips, bracing or casting may be required for some time postoperatively to maintain containment.[242] The proposed advantage of this approach is the ability to obtain greater coverage of the femoral head than is possible from either osteotomy alone.

Chiari Osteotomy

Although several authors report the use of Chiari's pelvic osteotomy as a primary procedure for Legg-Calvé-Perthes disease,[243-245] the most common use for the procedure is the healing femoral head that remains lateralized.[246,247] The Chiari procedure has been characterized by some authors as difficult, exacting, or dangerous.[248-250] Because the femoral head will often show gradual improvement in roundness until skeletal maturity even without treatment, the true effectiveness of this intervention remains unproven.[153] Bennett and associates[247] recommend this procedure for the older child with a painful hip, severe deformity of the femoral head, and incongruency of the femoral head and acetabulum demonstrated by arthrography.

Cheilectomy Excision of the extruded fragment of the femoral head, usually the anterolateral portion, has been recommended in the past by Garceau and associates.[251] This procedure has fallen out of favor and rarely is done today because of a number of devastating complications. The excision of the head fragment weakens the attachment of the head to the neck and can lead to a slip of the epiphysis, and the operation should never be done before closure of the capital physis. Stiffness is such a frequent complication of the procedure that it has been almost completely abandoned.[234]

Valgus Osteotomy Valgus osteotomy was recommended by Salter and associates[252] in 1978 and Catterall[94] in 1982 for a flattened femoral head that blocks abduction, a condition termed "hinge abduction" (Fig. 27). The procedure is recom-

mended if the hip is congruous in adduction, and if it will adduct further than the congruous position. Although the most obvious effect is to improve the gait by abducting the extremity, it has also been suggested that the femoral head may "round up" as a result of the procedure.[94] Quain and Catterall[253] reported improved range of motion, reduction of pain, improvement of limb length, improvement of joint space, healing of central head fragmentation, and reduction of subluxation in a series of 23 cases. There are no long-term studies of the effectiveness of the procedure.

Excision of Osteochondritic Fragment A few patients who have had Legg-Calvé-Perthes disease will develop pain in late adolescence after a long symptom-free period. When there are symptoms of locking, catching, or crepitation, an osteochondritic defect may be found in the femoral head (Figs. 20 and 21).[234,254] The diagnosis should be considered when radiographs show a lucent area in the central portion of the femoral head. It is often difficult to determine if the area is a loose fragment or just an area of softened cartilage and fibrous tissue. The diagnosis of a loose body can be confirmed by arthrography if the contrast material surrounds the lesion.[255,256] The absence of this finding does not, however, rule out a loose fragment, and it may be necessary to perform arthroscopy or arthrotomy of the hip to evaluate the lesion.[257]

If symptoms are not disabling, conservative management consisting of anti-inflammatory medication, rest, and avoidance of inciting activities may be successful. Kamhi and MacEwen[258] described seven cases with apparent osteochondritic defects and stated that nonsurgical management was usually successful. Bowen and associates[147] reported 14 of 465 cases of Legg-Calvé-Perthes disease, and only four required surgery. Osterman and Lindholm[146] followed 17 patients with apparent osteochondritic lesions for a mean of 32 years. Only three hips developed a loose body within the joint, and they concluded that most such hips could be managed without surgery.

When surgical removal is elected, the lesion may be visible during an arthrotomy with retraction of the joint, but it is often necessary to dislocate the hip to see the central fragment.[256,259] Arthroscopic excision of loose bodies has been successful, and it is recommended that the bed of the defect be debrided.[147,260] When there is a softened area in the femoral head without a loose fragment, the management is controversial. It may be helpful to drill such an area in an effort to stimulate vascular ingrowth and healing, but there are few data regarding this approach.

CONCLUSION

Legg-Calvé-Perthes disease is a fascinating disorder, which was discovered this century with the advent of the first modern machine directed toward the field of medicine. The disorder has now been studied pathologically, radiographically, ultrasonographically, scintigraphically, arthrographically, and with MRI. The genetics of the disease, its relationship to coagulopathy, to synovitis, to trauma, and to skeletal maturation have been studied. The susceptible child has been identified, and yet the exact cause of the disease is still unknown. It is suspected that this susceptible child may be more frequently traumatizing an immature femoral head, thereby causing an avascular event to occur. Perhaps the terminal branch of the circumflex artery is pinched in the cartilage of the edge of the femoral head. Or, perhaps, on the venous side of the circulation, the trauma sets up a thrombus that fails to be lysed because of a subtle abnormality of the clot lysis mechanism.

The result is an evolution of osteonecrosis that varies in severity with the extent of femoral head involvement and with the age and maturity of the child. Half of the affected children will do well without treatment, whereas the other half will develop problems sometime in adulthood. Orthopaedists believe that it is possible to radiographically identify, with some accuracy, those likely to have permanent femoral head deformation and that early containment treatment can improve the chances of a good outcome in those patients. The short-term aim of investigators and physicians dealing with this disorder is to clarify exactly what the best treatment is for a given child, when and how that treatment should be applied, and how quickly it can be withdrawn. The long-term aim is to be able to identify the susceptible child and to prevent him or her from developing the disorder.

REFERENCES

1. Goff CW (ed): *Legg-Calvé-Perthes Syndrome and Related Osteochondroses of Youth*. Springfield, IL, Charles C Thomas, 1954.

2. Legg AT: An obscure affection of the hip-joint. *Boston Med Surg J* 1910;162:202-204.

3. Calvé J: Sur une forme particuliére de pseudo-coxalgie greffée sur des déformations caractéristiques de l'extremité supérieure du fémur. *Rev Chir* 1910;30:54-84.

4. Calvé J: The classic: On a particular form of pseudo-coxalgia associated with a characteristic deformity of the upper end of the femur. *Clin Orthop* 1980;150:4-7.

5. Perthes G: Über Arthritis deformans juvenilis. *Deutsche Z Chir* 1910;107:111-159.

6. Waldenström H: Der obere tuberkulöse Collumherd. *Z Orthop Chir* 1909;24:487-512.

7. Legg AT: Osteochondral trophopathy of the hip-joint. *Surg Gynecol Obstet* 1916;22:307-323.

8. Freiberg AH: Coxa vara adolescentium and osteoarthritis deformans coxae. *Am J Orthop Surg* 1905;3:6-14.

9. Perthes G: Ueber osteochondritis deformans juvenilis. *Arch Klin Chir* 1913;101:779-807.

10. Schwarz E: Eire typische Erkrankung der oberen Femurepiphyse. *Beitr Klin Chir* 1914;93:1.

11. Calvé J, Galland M, de Cagny R: Pathogenesis of the limp due to coxalgia: The antalgic gait. *J Bone Joint Surg* 1939;21:12-25.

12. Perthes G: Osteochondritis deformans odor Legg's disease. *Zentralbl F Chir* 1920;47:123-125.

13. Herring JA: Legg-Calvé-Perthes disease: A review of current knowledge, in Barr JS Jr (ed): *Instructional Course Lectures XXXVIII*. Park Ridge, IL, American Academy of Orthopaedic Surgeons, 1989, pp 309-315.

14. Legg AT: The end results of coxa plana. *J Bone Joint Surg* 1927;9:26-36.

15. Waldenström H: On Coxa plana: Osteochondritis deformans coxae juvenilis. *Acta Chir Scand* 1923;55:577-590.

16. Pike MM: Legg-Perthes Disease: A method of conservative treatment. *J Bone Joint Surg* 1950;32A:663-670.

17. Goff CW: Influence of small daily doses of tetracycline on the clinical course of Legg-Calvé-Perthes syndrome: Report of a double-blind study. *Clin Orthop* 1965;38:71-80.

18. Snyder CH: A sling for use in Legg-Perthes disease. *J Bone Joint Surg* 1947;29:524-526.

19. Harrison MH, Menon MP: Legg-Calvé-Perthes disease: The value of roentgenographic measurement in clinical practice with special reference to the broomstick plaster method. *J Bone Joint Surg* 1966;48A:1301-1318.

20. Harrison MH, Turner MH, Nicholson FJ: Coxa Plana: Results of a new form of splinting. *J Bone Joint Surg* 1969;51A:1057-1069.

21. Eyre-Brook AL: Osteochondritis deformans coxae juvenilis or Perthes' disease: The results of treatment by traction in recumbency. *Br J Surg* 1936;24:166-182.

22. Salter RB: Legg-Perthes disease: The scientific basis for the methods of treatment and their indications. *Clin Orthop* 1980;150:8-11.

23. Burwell RG: Perthes' disease: Growth and aetiology. *Arch Dis Child* 1988;63:1408-1412.

24. Girdany BR, Osman MZ: Longitudinal growth and skeletal maturation in Perthes' disease. *Radiol Clin North Am* 1968;6:245-251.

25. Fisher RL: An epidemiological study of Legg-Perthes disease. *J Bone Joint Surg* 1972;54A:769-778.

26. Bohr HH: Skeletal maturation in Legg-Calvé-Perthes' disease. *Int Orthop* 1979;2:277-281.

27. Kristmundsdottir F, Burwell RG, Hall DJ, et al: A longitudinal study of carpal bone development in Perthes' disease: Its significance for both radiologic standstill and bilateral disease. *Clin Orthop* 1986;209:115-123.

28. Harrison MH, Turner MH, Jacobs P: Skeletal immaturity in Perthes' disease. *J Bone Joint Surg* 1976;58B:37-40.

29. Kristmundsdottir F, Burwell RG, Harrison MH: Delayed skeletal maturation in Perthes' disease. *Acta Orthop Scand* 1987;58:277-279.

30. Exner GU, Schreiber A: Growth retardation and compensatory growth in Perthes disease. *Z Orthop* 1986;124:192-195.

31. Cannon SR, Pozo JL, Catterall A: Elevated growth velocity in children with Perthes' disease. *J Pediatr Orthop* 1989;9:285-292.

32. Wynne-Davies R, Gormley J: The aetiology of Perthes' disease: Genetic, epidemiological and growth factors in 310 Edinburgh and Glasgow patients. *J Bone Joint Surg* 1978;60B:6-14.

33. Hall AJ, Barker DJ, Dangerfield PH, et al: Small feet and Perthes' disease: A survey in Liverpool. *J Bone Joint Surg* 1988;70B:611-613.

34. Tanaka H, Tamura K, Takano K, et al: Serum somatomedin A in Perthes' disease. *Acta Orthop Scand* 1984;55:135-140.

35. Motokawa S: Effect of serum factors on skeletal growth in Perthes' disease. *Nippon Seikeigeka Gakkai Zasshi* 1990;64:790-797.

36. Neidel J, Zander D, Hackenbroch MH: No physiologic age-related increase of circulating somatomedin-C during early stage of Perthes' disease: A longitudinal study in 21 boys. *Arch Orthop Trauma Surg* 1992;111:171-173.

37. Kitsugi T, Kasahara Y, Seto Y, et al: Normal somatomedin-C activity measured by radioimmunoassay in Perthes' disease. *Clin Orthop* 1989;244:217-221.

38. Neidel J, Boddenberg B, Zander D, et al: Thyroid function in Legg-Calvé-Perthes disease: Cross-sectional and longitudinal study. *J Pediatr Orthop* 1993;13:592-597.

39. Ponseti IV, Cotton RL: Legg-Calvé-Perthes disease: Pathogenesis and evolution: Failure of treatment with L-triiodothyronine. *J Bone Joint Surg* 1961;43A:261-274.

40. Rayner PH, Schwalbe SL, Hall DJ: An assessment of endocrine function in boys with Perthes' disease. *Clin Orthop* 1986;209:124-128.

41. Arie E, Johnson F, Harrison MH, et al: Femoral head shape in Perthes' disease: Is the contralateral hip abnormal? *Clin Orthop* 1986;209:77-88.

42. Harrison MH, Blakemore ME: A study of the "normal" hip in children with unilateral Perthes' disease. *J Bone Joint Surg* 1980;62B:31-36.

43. Ippolito E: Legg-Calvé-Perthes (L.C.P.) disease in the light of recent findings. *Ital J Orthop Traumatol* 1982;8:77-92.

44. Ponseti IV: Legg Pethes Disease: Observations on pathological changes in two cases. *J Bone Joint Surg* 1956;38A:739-750.

45. Harper PS, Brotherton BJ, Cochlin D: Genetic risks in Perthes' disease. *Clin Genet* 1976;10:178-182.

46. Hall DJ: Genetic aspects of Perthes' disease: A critical review. *Clin Orthop* 1986;209:100-114.

47. Burch PR, Nevelos AB: Perthes' disease: A new genetic hypothesis. *Med Hypotheses* 1979;5:513-528.

48. O'Sullivan M, O'Rourke SK, MacAuley P: Legg-Calvé-Perthes disease in a family: Genetic or environmental. *Clin Orthop* 1985;199:179-181.

49. Hall DJ, Harrison MH, Burwell RG: Congenital abnormalities and Perthes' disease: Clinical evidence that children with Perthes' disease may have a major congenital defect. *J Bone Joint Surg* 1979;61B:18-25.

50. Hall AJ, Barker DJ, Dangerfield PH, et al: Perthes' disease of the hip in Liverpool. *Br Med J* 1983;287:1757-1759.

51. Hall AJ, Barker DJ: Perthes' disease in Yorkshire. *J Bone Joint Surg* 1989;71B:229-233.

52. Hall AJ, Margetts BM, Barker DJ, et al: Low blood manganese levels in Liverpool children with Perthes' disease. *Paediatr Perinat Epidemiol* 1989;3:131-135.

53. Hall AJ, Barker DJ, Lawton D: The social origins of Perthes' disease of the hip. *Paediatr Perinat Epidemiol* 1990;4:64-70.

54. Douglas G, Rang M: The role of trauma in the pathogenesis of the osteochondroses. *Clin Orthop* 1981;158:28-32.

55. Chung SM: The arterial supply of the developing proximal end of the human femur. *J Bone Joint Surg* 1976;58A:961-970.

56. Loder RT, Schwartz EM, Hensinger RN: Behavioral characteristics of children with Legg-Calvé-Perthes disease. *J Pediatr Orthop* 1993;13:598-601.

57. Catterall A, Pringle J, Byers PD, et al: A review of the morphology of Perthes' disease. *J Bone Joint Surg* 1982;64B:269-275.

58. Inoue A, Freeman MA, Vernon-Roberts B, et al: The pathogenesis of Perthes' disease. *J Bone Joint Surg* 1976;58B:453-461.

59. Wingstrand H, Bauer GC, Brismar J, et al: Transient ischaemia of the proximal femoral epiphysis in the child: Interpretation of bone scintimetry for diagnosis in hip pain. *Acta Orthop Scand* 1985;56:197-203.

60. Rutskii AV, Kovalenko IuD, Kriuchok VV, et al: Dynamic angioscintigraphy and static scintigraphy of the hip joint in the complex diagnosis of Legg-Perthes disease. *Ortop Travmatol Protez* 1989;10:35-39.

61. Théron J: Angiography in Legg-Calvé-Perthes disease. *Radiology* 1980;135:81-92.

62. de Camargo FP, de Godoy RM Jr, Tovo R: Angiography in Perthes' disease. *Clin Orthop* 1984;191:216-220.

63. O'Hara JP III, Dommisse GF: Extraosseous blood supply to the neonatal femoral head. *Clin Orthop* 1983;174:293-297.

64. Fujikawa K: Comparative vascular anatomy of the hip of the miniature dog and of the normal-size mongrel. *Kurume Med J* 1991;38:159-165.

65. Liu SL, Ho TC: The role of venous hypertension in the pathogenesis of Legg-Perthes disease: A clinical and experimental study. *J Bone Joint Surg* 1991;73A:194-200.

66. Tao SN: Hemodynamics changes in proximal femur of patients with femoral head necrosis. *Chung Hua Nai Ko Tsa Chih* 1991;29:452-454,464.

67. Iwasaki K, Suzuki R, Okazaki T, et al: The haemodynamics of Perthes' disease: An intraosseous venographic study combined with measurement of the intramedullary pressure. *Int Orthop* 1982;6:141-148.

68. Suramo I, Vuoria P: Cineangiographic study of the venous drainage of the femoral neck in children. *Ann Clin Res* 1976;8:8-14.

69. Green NE, Griffin PP: Intra-osseous venous pressure in Legg-Perthes disease. *J Bone Joint Surg* 1982;64A:666-671.

70. Heikkinen E, Lanning P, Suramo I, et al: The venous drainage of the femoral neck as a prognostic sign in Perthes' disease. *Acta Orthop Scand* 1980;51:501-503.

71. Rand C, Pearson TC, Heatley FW: Avascular necrosis of the femoral head in sickle cell syndrome: A report of 5 cases. *Acta Haematol* 1987;78:186-192.

72. Ebong WW: Avascular necrosis of the femoral head associated with haemoglobinopathy. *Trop Geogr Med* 1977;29:19-23.

73. Orzincolo C, Castaldi G, Scutellari PN, et al: Aseptic necrosis of femoral head complicating thalassemia. *Skeletal Radiol* 1986;15:541-544.

74. Alabi ZO, Durosinmi MA: Legg-Calvé-Perthes' disease associated with chronic myeloid leukaemia in a child: Case report. *East Afr Med J* 1989;66:556-559.

75. Renowden S, Fitzgerald EJ, Kemp AM: Non-Hodgkin's lymphoma of bone causing avascular necrosis of the femoral head. *Postgrad Med J* 1988;64:68-70.

76. Pettersson H, Wingstrand H, Thambert C: Legg-Calvé-Perthes disease in hemophilia: Incidence and etiologic considerations. *J Pediatr Orthop* 1990;10:28-32.

77. Ura Y, Hara T, Mori Y, et al: Development of Perthes' disease in a 3-year-old boy with idiopathic thrombocytopenic purpura and antiphospholipid antibodies. *Pediatr Hematol Oncol* 1992;9:77-80.

78. Kleinman RG, Bleck EE: Increased blood viscosity in patients with Legg-Perthes disease: A preliminary report. *J Pediatr Orthop* 1981;1:131-136.

79. Glueck CJ, Glueck HI, Greenfield D, et al: Protein C and S deficiency, thrombophilia, and hypofibrinolysis: Pathophysiologic causes of Legg-Perthes disease. *Pediatr Res* 1994;35:383-388.

80. Glueck CJ, Crawford A, Roy D, et al: Association of antithrombotic factor deficiencies and hypofibrinolysis with Legg-Perthes disease. *J Bone Joint Surg* 1996;78A:3-13.

81. Kallio P, Ryöppy S, Kunnamo I: Transient synovitis and Perthes' disease: Is there an aetiological connection? *J Bone Joint Surg* 1986;68B:808-811.

82. Sharwood PF: The irritable hip syndrome in children: A long-term follow-up. *Acta Orthop Scand* 1981;52:633-638.

83. Mukamel M, Litmanovitch M, Yosipovich Z, et al: Legg-Calvé-Perthes disease following transient synovitis: How often? *Clin Pediatr* 1985;24:629-631.

84. Haueisen DC, Weiner DS, Weiner SD: The characterization of "transient synovitis of the hip" in children. *J Pediatr Orthop* 1986;6:11-17.

85. Landin LA, Danielson LG, Wattsgard G: Transient synovitis of the hip: Its incidence, epidemiology, and relation to Perthes' disease. *J Bone Joint Surg* 1987;69B:238-242.

86. Mallet JF, Rigault P, Padovani JP, et al: Transient synovitis of the hip in childhood: "Observation hip." *Rev Chir Orthop Reparatrice Appar Mot* 1981;67:791-803.

87. Pay NT, Singer WS, Bartal E: Hip pain in three children accompanied by transient abnormal findings on MR images. *Radiology* 1989;171:147-149.

88. Houben JJ, Godart S, Abramovic J, et al: Vascular disorders in irritable hip disclosed by dynamic scintigraphy with radioactive colloids. *Chir Pediatr* 1982;23:309-314.

89. Glefand MJ, Ball WS, Oestreich AE, et al: Transient loss of femoral head Tc-99m diphosphonate uptake with prolonged maintenance of femoral head architecture. *Clin Nucl Med* 1983;8:347-354.

90. Vegter J: The influence of joint posture on intra-articular pressure: A study of transient synovitis and Perthes' disease. *J Bone Joint Surg* 1987;69B:71-74.

91. Kallio P, Ryöppy S: Hyperpressure in juvenile hip disease. *Acta Orthop Scand* 1985;56:211-214.

92. Ponseti IV, Maynard JA, Weinstein SL, et al: Legg-Calvé-Perthes disease: Histochemical and ultrastructural observations of the epiphyseal cartilage and physis. *J Bone Joint Surg* 1983;65A:797-807.

93. Mickelson MR, McCurnin DM, Awbrey BJ, et al: Legg-Calvé-Perthes disease in dogs: A comparison to human Legg-Calvé-Perthes disease. *Clin Orthop* 1981;157:287-300.

94. Catterall A (ed): *Legg-Calvé-Perthes' Disease*. Edinburgh, Scotland, Churchill-Livingstone, 1982.

95. Waldenström H: The definite form of the coxa plana. *Acta Radiologica* 1922;1:384-394.

96. Herring JA, Neustadt JB, Williams JJ, et al: The lateral pillar classification of Legg-Calvé-Perthes disease. *J Pediatr Orthop* 1992;12:143-150.

97. Salter RB, Thompson GH: Legg-Calvé-Perthes disease: The prognostic significance of the subchondral fracture and a two-group classification of the femoral head involvement. *J Bone Joint Surg* 1984;66A:479-489.

98. Roy DR: Perthes'-like changes caused by acquired hypothyroidism. *Orthopedics* 1991;14:901-904.

99. Daudet M, David M, Aimard P: Lesions of the hip in congenital myxedema in children. *Chir Pediatr* 1986;27:94-99.

100. Mandell GA, Harcke HT, Kumar SJ: Avascular necrosis and related conditions. *Top Magn Reson Imaging* 1991;4:31-44.

101. Andersen PE Jr, Schantz K, Bollerslev J, et al: Bilateral femoral head dysplasia and osteochondritis: Multiple epiphyseal dysplasia tarda, spondylo-epiphyseal dysplasia tarda, and bilateral Legg-Perthes disease. *Acta Radiol* 1988;29:705-709.

102. Crossan JF, Wynne-Davies R, Fulford GE: Bilateral failure of the capital femoral epiphysis: Bilateral Perthes disease, multiple epiphyseal dysplasia, pseudoachondroplasia, and spondyloepiphyseal dysplasia congenita and tarda. *J Pediatr Orthop* 1983;3:297-301.

103. Ikegawa S, Nagano A, Nakamura K: A case of multiple epiphyseal dysplasia complicated by unilateral Perthes' disease. *Acta Orthop Scand* 1991;62:606-608.

104. Mandell GA, MacKenzie WG, Scott CI Jr, et al: Identification of avascular necrosis in the dysplastic proximal femoral epiphysis. *Skeletal Radiol* 1989;18:273-281.

105. Paterson DE, Harper G, Weston HJ, et al: Maroteaux-Lamy syndrome, mild form: MPS vi b. *Br J Radiol* 1982;55:805-812.

106. Bowen JR, Schmidt T: Osteochondroma of the femoral neck in Perthes disease. *J Pediatr Orthop* 1983;3:28-30.

107. Katz JF: Osteochondroma of the neck of the femur in Legg-Calvé-Perthes disease: Report of two cases. *Clin Orthop* 1970;68:50-54.

108. Milgram JW: Synovial osteochondromatosis in association with Legg-Calvé-Perthes disease. *Clin Orthop* 1979;145:179-182.

109. Keret D, Bassett GS: Avascular necrosis of the capital femoral epiphysis in metachondromatosis. *J Pediatr Orthop* 1990;10:658-661.

110. Pfeiffer RA, Bauer H, Petersen C: The Schwartz-Jampel syndrome (myotonia chondrodystrophica). *Helv Paediatr Acta* 1977;32:251-261.

111. Howell CJ, Wynne-Davies R: The tricho-rhino-phalangeal syndrome: A report of 14 cases in 7 kindreds. *J Bone Joint Surg* 1986;68B:311-314.

112. Verbruggen LA, Van Laere C, Lamoureux J, et al: Tricho-rhino-phalangeal syndrome type I in a Belgian family. *Clin Rheumatol* 1987;6:185-191.

113. Stearns ZR, Lacassie Y, MacEwen GD: Perthes-like disease and the tricho-rhino-phalangeal syndromes: The first black patient. *Orthopedics* 1990;13:468-473.

114. Herold HZ: Avascular necrosis of the femoral head in children under the age of three. *Clin Orthop* 1977;126:193-195.

115. Graziano GP, Kernek CB, DeRosa GP: Coexistent Legg-Calvé-Perthes disease and slipped capital femoral epiphysis in the same child. *J Pediatr Orthop* 1987;7:61-62.

116. Barquet A: Natural history of avascular necrosis following traumatic hip dislocation in childhood: A review of 145 cases. *Acta Orthop Scand* 1982;53:815-820.

117. Ozonoff MB, Ziter FM Jr: The femoral head notch. *Skeletal Radiol* 1987;16:19-22.

118. Gower WE, Johnston RC: Legg-Perthes disease: Long-term follow-up of thirty-six patients. *J Bone Joint Surg* 1971;53A:759-768.

119. Moller PF: The clinical observations after healing of Calvé-Perthes' disease compared with the final deformities left by that disease, and the bearing of those final deformities on the ultimate prognosis. *Acta Radiol* 1926;5:1-36.

120. Brotherton BJ, McKibbin B: Perthes' disease treated by prolonged recumbency and femoral head containment: A long-term appraisal. *J Bone Joint Surg* 1977;59B:8-14.

121. Evans IK, Deluca PA, Gage JR: A comparative study of ambulation-abduction bracing and varus derotation osteotomy in the treatment of severe Legg-Calvé-Perthes disease in children over 6 years of age. *J Pediatr Orthop* 1988;8:676-682.

122. Hoikka V, Lindholm TS, Poussa M: Intertrochanteric varus osteotomy in Legg-Calvé-Perthes disease: A report of 112 hips. *J Pediatr Orthop* 1986;6:600-604.

123. Ingman AM, Paterson DC, Sutherland AD: A comparison between innominate osteotomy and hip spica in the treatment of Legg-Perthes' disease. *Clin Orthop* 1982;163:141-147.

124. Catterall A: The natural history of Perthes' disease. *J Bone Joint Surg* 1971;53B:37-53.

125. Hardcastle PH, Ross R, Hamalainen M, et al: Catterall grouping of Perthes' disease: An assessment of observer error and prognosis using the Catterall classification. *J Bone Joint Surg* 1980;62B:428-431.

126. Christensen F, Soballe K, Ejsted R, et al: The Catterall classification of Perthes' disease: An assessment of reliability. *J Bone Joint Surg* 1986;68B:614-615.

127. Van Dam BE, Crider RJ, Noyes JD, et al: Determination of the Catterall classification in Legg-Calvé-Perthes disease. *J Bone Joint Surg* 1981;63A:906-914.

128. Dickens DR, Menelaus MB: The assessment of prognosis in Perthes' disease. *J Bone Joint Surg* 1978;60B:189-194.

129. Poussa M, Hoikka V, Yrjonen T, et al: Early signs of poor prognosis in Legg-Perthes-Calvé disease treated by femoral varus osteotomy. *Rev Chir Orthop Reparatrice Appar Mot* 1991;77:478-482.

130. Mukherjee A, Fabry G: Evaluation of the prognostic indices in Legg-Calvé-Perthes disease: Statistical analysis of 116 hips. *J Pediatr Orthop* 1990;10:153-158.

131. Yrjonen T, Poussa M, Hoikka V, et al: Poor prognosis in atypical Perthes' disease: Radiographic analysis of 19 hips after 35 years. *Acta Orthop Scand* 1992;63:399-402.

132. Ferguson AB Jr: Pathology and treatment of Legg-Perthes disease. *Pediatr Ann* 1976;5:113-129.

133. Rab GT, Wyatt M, Sutherland DH, et al: A technique for determining femoral head containment during gait. *J Pediatr Orthop* 1985;5:8-12.

134. Ritterbusch JF, Shantharam SS, Gelinas C: Comparison of lateral pillar classification and Catterall classification of Legg-Calvé-Perthes' disease. *J Pediatr Orthop* 1993;13:200-202.

135. Mose K: Methods of measuring in Legg-Calvé-Perthes disease with special regard to the prognosis. *Clin Orthop* 1980;150:103-109.

136. Stulberg SD, Cooperman DR, Wallensten R: The natural history of Legg-Calvé-Perthes disease. *J Bone Joint Surg* 1981;63A:1095-1108.

137. Helbo S (ed): *Morbus Calvé-Perthes*. Odense, Denmark, Fyns Tidendes Bogtrykkeri, 1953.

138. Eaton GO: Long-term results of treatment in coxa plana: A follow-up study of eighty-eight patients. *J Bone Joint Surg* 1967;49A:1031-1042.

139. Ratliff AH: Perthes' disease: A study of thirty-four hips observed for thirty years. *J Bone Joint Surg* 1967;49B:102-107.

140. Engelhardt P: Late prognosis of Perthes' disease: Which factors determine arthritis risk? *Z Orthop* 1985;123:168-181.

141. Saito S, Takaoka K, Ono K, et al: Residual deformities related to arthrotic change after Perthes' disease: A long-term follow-up of fifty-one cases. *Arch Orthop Trauma Surg* 1985;104:7-14.

142. Perpich M, McBeath A, Kruse D: Long-term follow-up of Perthes disease treated with spica casts. *J Pediatr Orthop* 1983;3:160-165.

143. McAndrew MP, Weinstein SL: A long-term follow-up of Legg-Calvé-Perthes disease. *J Bone Joint Surg* 1984;66A:860-869.

144. Snyder CR: Legg-Perthes disease in the young hip: Does it necessarily do well? *J Bone Joint Surg* 1975;57A:751-759.

145. Ippolito E, Tudisco C, Farsetti P: Long-term prognosis of Legg-Calvé-Perthes disease developing during adolescence. *J Pediatr Orthop* 1985;5:652-656.

146. Osterman K, Lindholm TS: Osteochondritis dissecans following Perthes' disease. *Clin Orthop* 1980;152:247-254.

147. Bowen JR, Kumar VP, Joyce JJ III, et al: Osteochondritis dissecans following Perthes' disease: Arthroscopic-operative treatment. *Clin Orthop* 1986;209:49-56.

148. Shapiro F: Legg-Calvé-Perthes disease: A study of lower extremity length discrepancies and skeletal maturation. *Acta Orthop Scand* 1982;53:437-444.

149. Solomon L: Patterns of osteoarthritis of the hip. *J Bone Joint Surg* 1976;58B:176-183.

150. Harris WH: Etiology of osteoarthritis of the hip. *Clin Orthop* 1986;213:20-33.

151. Cooperman DR, Emery H, Keller C: Factors relating to hip joint arthritis following three childhood diseases: Juvenile rheumatoid arthritis, Perthes disease, and postreduction avascular necrosis in congenital hip dislocation. *J Pediatr Orthop* 1986;6:706-712.

152. Clarke NM, Harrison MH: Painful sequelae of coxa plana. *J Bone Joint Surg* 1983;65A:13-18.

153. Herring JA, Williams JJ, Neustadt JN, et al: Evolution of femoral head deformity during the healing phase of Legg-Calvé-Perthes disease. *J Pediatr Orthop* 1993;13:41-45.

154. Weinstein SL: Legg-Calvé-Perthes disease, in Morrissy RT (ed): *Pediatric Orthopaedics,* ed 3. Philadelphia, PA, JB Lippincott, 1990, vol 2, pp 851-883.

155. Waldenström H: The first stages of coxa plana. *J Bone Joint Surg* 1938;20A:559-566.

156. Caffey J: The early roentgenographic changes in essential coxa plana: Their significance in pathogenesis. *Am J Roentgenol* 1968;103:620-634.

157. Kamegaya M: Comparative study of Perthes' disease treated by various ambulatory orthoses. *Nippon Seikeigeka Gakkai Zasshi* 1987;61:917-932.

158. Ferguson AB Jr: The pathology of Legg-Perthes disease and its comparison with aseptic necrosis. *Clin Orthop* 1975;106:7-18.

159. Brown I: A study of the "capsular" shadow in disorders of the hip in children. *J Bone Joint Surg* 1975;57B:175-179.

160. Nevelös AB: Bilateral Perthes' disease. *Acta Orthop Scand* 1980;51:649-654.

161. Gill AB: Legg-Perthes disease of the hip: Its early roentgenographic manifestations and its cyclical course. *J Bone Joint Surg* 1940;22A:1013-1047.

162. Ponseti IV: Legg-Perthes disease: Observations on pathological changes in two cases. *J Bone Joint Surg* 1956;38A:739-750.

163. Katz JF, Siffert RS: Capital necrosis, metaphyseal cyst and subluxation in coxa plana. *Clin Orthop* 1975;106:75-85.

164. Hoffinger SA, Henderson RC, Renner JB, et al: Magnetic resonance evaluation of "metaphyseal" changes in Legg-Calvé-Perthes disease. *J Pediatr Orthop* 1993;13:602-606.

165. Hoffinger SA, Rab GT, Salamon PB: "Metaphyseal" cysts in Legg-Calvé-Perthes' disease. *J Pediatr Orthop* 1991;11:301-306.

166. Aguirre M, Pellise F, Castellote A: Metaphyseal cysts in Legg-Calvé-Perthes disease. *J Pediatr Orthop* 1992;12:404-405.

167. Apley AG, Wientroub S: The sagging rope sign in Perthes' disease and allied disorders. *J Bone Joint Surg* 1981;63B:43-47.

168. Keret D, Harrison MH, Clarke NM, et al: Coxa plana: The fate of the physis. *J Bone Joint Surg* 1984;66A:870-877.

169. Barnes JM: Premature epiphysial closure in Perthes' disease. *J Bone Joint Surg* 1980;62B:432-437.

170. Bowen JR, Schreiber FC, Foster BK, et al: Premature femoral neck physeal closure in Perthes' disease. *Clin Orthop* 1982;171:24-29.

171. Sponseller PD, Desai SS, Millis MB: Abnormalities of proximal femoral growth after severe Perthes' disease. *J Bone Joint Surg* 1989;71B:610-614.

172. Langenskiöld A: Changes in the capital growth plate and the proximal femoral metaphysis in Legg-Calvé-Perthes disease. *Clin Orthop* 1980;150:110-114.

173. Yngve DA, Roberts JM: Acetabular hypertrophy in Legg-Calvé-Perthes disease. *J Pediatr Orthop* 1985;5:416-421.

174. Joseph B: Morphological changes in the acetabulum in Perthes' disease. *J Bone Joint Surg* 1989;71B:756-763.

175. Kamegaya M, Shinada Y, Moriya H, et al: Acetabular remodelling in Perthes' disease after primary healing. *J Pediatr Orthop* 1992;12:308-314.

176. Meyer J: Dysplasia epiphysealis capitis femoris: A clinical radiological syndrome and its relationship to Legg-Calvé-Perthes disease. *Acta Orthop Scand* 1964;34:183-197.

177. Herring JA, Lundeen MA, Wenger DR: Minimal Perthes' disease. *J Bone Joint Surg* 1980;62B:25-30.

178. Axer A, Schiller MG: The pathogenesis of the early deformity of the capital femoral epiphysis in Legg-Calvé-Perthes syndrome (L.C.P.S.): An arthrographic study. *Clin Orthop* 1972;84:106-115.

179. Gershuni DH, Axer A, Hendel D: Arthrographic findings in Legg-Calvé-Perthes disease and transient synovitis of the hip. *J Bone Joint Surg* 1978;60A:457-464.

180. Crawford AH, Carothers TA: Hip arthrography in the skeletally immature. *Clin Orthop* 1982;162:54-60.

181. Gallagher JM, Weiner DS, Cook AJ: When is arthrography indicated in Legg-Calvé-Perthes disease? *J Bone Joint Surg* 1983;65A:900-905.

182. Suzuki S, Awaya G, Okada Y, et al: Examination by ultrasound of Legg-Calvé-Perthes disease. *Clin Orthop* 1987;220:130-136.

183. Naumann T, Kollmannsberger A, Fischer M, et al: Ultrasonographic evaluation of Legg-Calvé-Perthes disease based on sonoanatomic criteria and the application of new measuring techniques. *Eur J Radiol* 1992;15:101-106.

184. Fasting OJ, Bjerkreim I, Langeland N, et al: Scintigraphic evaluation of the severity of Perthes' disease in the initial stage. *Acta Orthop Scand* 1980;51:655-660.

185. Oshima M, Yoshihasi Y, Ito K, et al: Initial stage of Legg-Calvé-Perthes disease: Comparison of three-phase bone scintigraphy and SPECT with MR imaging. *Eur J Radiol* 1992;15:107-112.

186. Conway JJ: A scintigraphic classification of Legg-Calvé-Perthes disease. *Semin Nucl Med* 1993;23:274-295.

187. Pinto MR, Peterson HA, Berquist TH: Magnetic resonance imaging in early diagnosis of Legg-Calvé-Perthes disease. *J Pediatr Orthop* 1989;9:19-22.

188. Theissen P, Rutt J, Linden A, et al: The early diagnosis of Perthes disease: The value of bone scintigraphy and magnetic resonance imaging in comparison with x-ray findings. *Nuklearmedizin* 1991;30:265-271.

189. Elsig PJ, Exner GU, von Schulthess GK, et al: False-negative magnetic resonance imaging in the early stage of Legg-Calvé-Perthes disease. *J Pediatr Orthop* 1989;9:231-235.

190. Scoles PV, Yoon YS, Makley JT, et al: Nuclear magnetic resonance imaging in Legg-Calvé-Perthes disease. *J Bone Joint Surg* 1984;66A:1357-1363.

191. Grimm J, Haist J, Higer HP: Diagnosis of Perthes disease using magnetic resonance tomography. *Z Orthop* 1991;129:151-155.

192. Ranner G, Ebner F, Fotter R, et al: Magnetic resonance imaging in children with acute hip pain. *Pediatr Radiol* 1989;20:67-71.

193. Henderson RC, Renner JB, Sturdivant MC, et al: Evaluation of magnetic resonance imaging in Legg-Perthes disease: A prospective, blinded study. *J Pediatr Orthop* 1990;10:289-297.

194. Egund N, Wingstrand H: Legg-Calvé-Perthes disease: Imaging with MR. *Radiology* 1991;179:89-92.

195. Bos CF, Bloem JL, Bloem RM: Sequential magnetic resonance imaging in Perthes' disease. *J Bone Joint Surg* 1991;73B:219-224.

196. Kumasaka Y, Watanabe H, Higashihara T, et al: Changes in the cartilaginous contour of Legg-Calvé-Perthes disease: Calculation on T1-weighted MR images. *Nippon Igaku Hoshasen Gakkai Zasshi* 1991;51:1232-1239.

197. Lee DY, Choi IH, Lee CK, et al: Assessment of complex hip deformity using three-dimensional CT image. *J Pediatr Orthop* 1991;11:13-19.

198. Weisz I, Bialik V, Adler O, et al: Some observations on the use of computerised tomography in Legg-Calvé-Perthes' disease. *Z Kinderchir* 1988;43:402-404.

199. Moreno P, Cahuzac JP, Pasquie M: Topographic and developmental study of primary osteochondritis of the hip by x-ray computed tomography. *Rev Chir Orthop Reparatrice Appar Mot* 1986;72:173-182.

200. Serlo W, Heikkinen E, Puranen J: Preoperative Russell traction in Legg-Calvé-Perthes disease. *J Pediatr Orthop* 1987;7:288-290.

201. Naito M, Schoenecker PL, Owen JH, et al: Acute effect of traction, compression, and hip joint tamponade on blood flow of the femoral head: An experimental model. *J Orthop Res* 1992;10:800-806.

202. Salter RB: Experimental and clinical aspects of Perthes' disease. *J Bone Joint Surg* 1966;48B:393-394.

203. Salter RB, Bell M: The pathogenesis of deformity in Legg-Perthes' disease: An experimental investigation. *J Bone Joint Surg* 1968;50B:436.

204. Rab GT: Determination of femoral head containment during gait. *Biomater Med Devices Artif Organs* 1983;11:31-38.

205. Reimers J: Incidence of full containment of the femoral head after Legg-Calvé-Perthes disease and in the "normal" hip. *J Pediatr Orthop* 1985;5:199-201.

206. Reimers J: The stability of the hip in children: A radiological study of the results of muscle surgery in cerebral palsy. *Acta Orthop Scand Suppl* 1980;184:1-100.

207. Petrie JG, Bitenc I: The abduction weight-bearing treatment in Legg-Perthes' disease. *J Bone Joint Surg* 1971;53B:54-62.

208. Richards BS, Coleman SS: Subluxation of the femoral head in coxa plana. *J Bone Joint Surg* 1987;69A:1312-1318.

209. Harrison MH, Turner MH, Smith DN: Perthes' disease: Treatment with the Birmingham splint. *J Bone Joint Surg* 1982;64B:3-11.

210. Bobechko WP, McLaurin CA, Motloch WM: Toronto orthosis for Legg-Perthes disease. *Artif Limbs* 1968;12:36-41.

211. Bobechko WP: The Toronto brace for Legg-Perthes disease. *Clin Orthop* 1974;102:115-117.

212. Drennan JC: Orthotic management of Legg-Perthes disease, in Leach RE, Hoaglund FT, Riseborough EJ (eds): *Controversies in Orthopaedic Surgery.* Philadelphia, PA, WB Saunders, 1982, pp 315-325.

213. Curtis BH, Gunther SF, Gossling HR, et al: Treatment for Legg-Perthes disease with the Newington ambulation-abduction brace. *J Bone Joint Surg* 1974;56A:1135-1146.

214. Roberts JM: Management of Legg-Calvé-Perthes syndrome in an ambulatory abduction brace. Proceedings of the First International Symposium on Legg-Calvé-Perthes Disease. Los Angeles, CA, Orthopaedic Hospital, 1977, pp 99-102.

215. Tachdjian MO, Jouett LD: Trilateral socket hip abduction orthosis for the treatment of Legg-Perthes disease. *J Bone Joint Surg* 1968; 50A:1272-1273.

216. Purvis JM, Dimon JH III, Meehan PL, et al: Preliminary experience with the Scottish Rite Hospital abduction orthosis for Legg-Perthes disease. *Clin Orthop* 1980;150:49-53.

217. Axer A: Subtrochanteric osteotomy in the treatment of Perthes' disease. *J Bone Joint Surg* 1965;47B:489-499.

218. Craig WA, Kramer WG, Watanabe R: Etiology and treatment of Legg-Calvé-Perthes syndrome. *J Bone Joint Surg* 1963;45A:1325-1326.

219. Lloyd-Roberts GC, Catterall A, Salamon PB: A controlled study of the indications for and the results of femoral osteotomy in Perthes' disease. *J Bone Joint Surg* 1976;58B:31-36.

220. McElwain JP, Regan BF, Dowling F, et al: Derotation varus osteotomy in Perthes disease. *J Pediatr Orthop* 1985;5:195-198.

221. Killian JT, Niemann KM: Preoperative skeletal traction in Legg-Perthes disease. *South Med J* 1985;78:928-932.

222. Clancy M, Steel HH: The effect of an incomplete intertrochanteric osteotomy on Legg-Calvé-Perthes disease. *J Bone Joint Surg* 1985;67A:213-216.

223. Kendig RJ, Evans GA: Biologic osteotomy in Perthes disease. *J Pediatr Orthop* 1986;6:278-284.

224. Marklund T, Tillberg B: Coxa plana: A radiological comparison of the rate of healing with conservative measures and after osteotomy. *J Bone Joint Surg* 1976;58B:25-30.

225. Karpinski MR, Newton G, Henry AP: The results and morbidity of varus osteotomy for Perthes' disease. *Clin Orthop* 1986;209:30-40.

226. Heikkinen E, Puranen J: Evaluation of femoral osteotomy in the treatment of Legg-Calvé-Perthes disease. *Clin Orthop* 1980;150:60-68.

227. Weiner SD, Weiner DS, Riley PM: Pitfalls in treatment of Legg-Calvé-Perthes disease using proximal femoral varus osteotomy. *J Pediatr Orthop* 1991;11:20-24.

228. Menelaus MB: Lessons learned in the management of Legg-Calvé-Perthes disease. *Clin Orthop* 1986;209:41-48.

229. Laurent LE, Poussa M: Intertrochanteric varus osteotomy in the treatment of Perthes' disease. *Clin Orthop* 1980;150:73-77.

230. Sponseller PD, Desai SS, Millis MB: Comparison of femoral and innominate osteotomies for the treatment of Legg-Calvé-Perthes disease. *J Bone Joint Surg* 1988;70A:1131-1139.

231. Leitch JM, Paterson DC, Foster BK: Growth disturbance in Legg-Calvé-Perthes disease and the consequences of surgical treatment. *Clin Orthop* 1991;262:178-184.

232. Axer A, Gershuni DH, Hendel D, et al: Indications for femoral osteotomy in Legg-Calvé-Perthes disease. *Clin Orthop* 1980;150:78-87.

233. Wenger DR: Selective surgical containment for Legg-Perthes disease: Recognition and management of complications. *J Pediatr Orthop* 1981;1:153-160.

234. Salter RB: The present status of surgical treatment for Legg-Perthes disease. *J Bone Joint Surg* 1984;66A:961-966.

235. Kalamchi A: Modified Salter osteotomy. *J Bone Joint Surg* 1982;64A:183-187.

236. Kehl DK, Coleman SS: An evaluation of Perthes' disease: Comparison of nonsurgical and surgical treatment. *Orthop Trans* 1981;5:407.

237. Kruse RW, Guille JT, Bowen JR: Shelf arthroplasty in patients who have Legg-Calvé-Perthes disease: A study of long-term results. *J Bone Joint Surg* 1991;73A:1338-1347.

238. Willett K, Hudson I, Catterall A: Lateral shelf acetabuloplasty: An operation for older children with Perthes' disease. *J Pediatr Orthop* 1992;12:563-568.

239. Gill AB: Plastic construction of an acetabulum in congenital dislocation of the hip: The shelf operation. *J Bone Joint Surg* 1935;17A:48-59.

240. Staheli LT, Chew DE: Slotted acetabular augmentation in childhood and adolescence. *J Pediatr Orthop* 1992;12:569-580.

241. Olney BW, Asher MA: Combined innominate and femoral osteotomy for the treatment of severe Legg-Calvé-Perthes disease. *J Pediatr Orthop* 1985;5:645-651.

242. Crutcher JP, Staheli LT: Combined osteotomy as a salvage procedure for severe Legg-Calvé-Perthes disease. *J Pediatr Orthop* 1992;12:151-156.

243. Cahuzac JP, Onimus M, Trottmann F, et al: Chiari pelvic osteotomy in Perthes disease. *J Pediatr Orthop* 1990;10:163-166.

244. Lack W, Feldner-Busztin H, Ritschl P, et al: The results of surgical treatment for Perthes' disease. *J Pediatr Orthop* 1989;9:197-204.

245. Chiari K: Medial displacement osteotomy of the pelvis. *Clin Orthop* 1974;98:55-71.

246. Klisic P, Bauer R, Bensahel H, et al: Chiari's pelvic osteotomy in the treatment of Legg-Calvé-Perthes disease. *Bull Hosp Jt Dis Orthop Inst* 1985;45:111-118.

247. Bennett JT, Mazurek RT, Cash JD: Chiari's osteotomy in the treatment of Perthes' disease. *J Bone Joint Surg* 1991;73B:225-228.

248. Bailey TE Jr, Hall JE: Chiari medial displacement osteotomy. *J Pediatr Orthop* 1985;5:635-641.

249. Benson MK, Evans DC: The pelvic osteotomy of Chiari: An anatomical study of the hazards and misleading radiographic appearances. *J Bone Joint Surg* 1976;58B:164-168.

250. DeWaal Malefijt MC, Hoogland T, Nielsen HK: Chiari osteotomy in the treatment of congenital dislocation and subluxation of the hip. *J Bone Joint Surg* 1982;64A:996-1004.

251. Garceau G, Rapp G, Lidge RT: Coxa plana (A surgical approach). *J Bone Joint Surg* 1973;55A:1313.

252. Salter RB, Willis R, Malcolm B: The treatment of residual subluxation and coxa vara by combined innominate osteotomy and abduction femoral osteotomy. *Ann Roy Coll Phys Surg Canada* 1978;63:11.

253. Quain S, Catterall A: Hinge abduction of the hip: Diagnosis and treatment. *J Bone Joint Surg* 1986;68B:61-64.

254. Grossbard GD: Hip pain during adolescence after Perthes' disease. *J Bone Joint Surg* 1981;63B:572-574.

255. Goldman AB, Hallel T, Salvati EM, et al: Osteochondritis dissecans complicating Legg-Perthes disease: A report of four cases. *Radiology* 1976;121:561-566.

256. Hallel T, Salvati EA: Osteochondritis dissecans following Legg-Calvé-Perthes disease: Report of three cases. *J Bone Joint Surg* 1976;58A:708-711.

257. Glick JM: Hip arthroscopy using the lateral approach, in Bassett FH III (ed): *Instructional Course Lectures XXXVII*. Park Ridge, IL, American Academy of Orthopaedic Surgeons, 1988, pp 223-231.

258. Kamhi E, MacEwen GD: Osteochondritis dissecans in Legg-Calvé-Perthes disease. *J Bone Joint Surg* 1975;57A:506-509.

259. Wood JB, Klassen RA, Peterson HA: Osteochondritis dissecans of the femoral head in children and adolescents: A report of 17 cases. *J Pediatr Orthop* 1995;15:313-316.

260. Schindler A, Lechevallier JJ, Rao NS, et al: Diagnostic and therapeutic arthroscopy of the hip in children and adolescents: Evaluation of results. *J Pediatr Orthop* 1995;15:317-321.

INDEX